HEALTH IS FOR EVERYBODY:

THE SCIENCE OF GETTING BETTER

WYATT PALUMBO

Health is for Everybody:

The Science of Getting Better

By Wyatt Palumbo,

Foreword by Howard Rankin PhD

Part I: The Body's DNA

Part II. Working Genetic Patterns

Part III. Shaping Your Own DNA

Part IV. Getting Better

__Foreword__

By Published Author and Psychologist, Dr. Howard Rankin

We are at a critical period in healthcare. As the science begins to reveal the truth about the body and mind, longstanding debates and concepts can finally be settled.

We now know that our body can cause symptoms in our mind and that our mind can cause symptoms in our bodies. That our bodies and minds aren't separate, but act as one cohesive unit.

We know that we have trillions of cells. And that these cells fire trillions of time every second, coming together to seamlessly manage our everyday life – like a trillion piece symphony acting in harmony for as long as we live.

Throughout my career, I have personally watched how childhoods shape intimate relationships. I have seen people whose choices culminate into struggle and despair.

I also know several people who were all told they had a few months to live, and every one of them defied that prognosis and all currently lead productive lives, decades after receiving their fatal prognosis.

With chronic illness posing one of the greatest modern threats to our health and well-being, it's time we all change our mindset about health, illness and our medical care. From our lifestyle to the tiniest of cells to our behaviors, environments, and upbringings – all of it matters to our health and quality of life.

Over my decades as a psychologist and now as an author and forever student of life – it is so clear to me that our bodies intuitively know how to heal. They are designed to optimize well-being and function and defend themselves in the best way possible. Our body is our ultimate guide through life.

It is also abundantly clear to me that at one point or another, it falls on us to know how to use it. No matter your circumstances, at some point your health will be your responsibility.

In this much needed book, Wyatt Palumbo combines these latest scientific discoveries with his own experiences and clinical methods into a simple to follow roadmap to not just feeling better, but being better.

From chronic pain and fatigue to multifaceted neurological and movement disorders, he and his team have seen some of the most complex chronic illnesses cases from around the country, having helped thousands take back their quality of life.

It's as clear to him as it is to me – your quality of life is more in your control than you think. That no matter your DNA, no matter your illness or circumstances – you *can* feel better. You *can* heal.

~Howard Rankin PhD

Part I: The Body's DNA

Nearly fifteen years ago, I was working as a medical intern in a healthcare clinic. I found myself in front of John. He came for help for his opiate use that began with an injury and had now ballooned into a full-blown addiction of 800mg of oxycodone per day.

I remember looking over to the managing physician at the time, stating the obvious – "he should have gone into withdrawal already."

I asked if the medication would be administered anyway and the doctor looked back and said, "He has to be in withdrawal from his oxycodone."

But John never went into withdrawal. Nothing was changing. His heart rate, blood pressure, pupils, temperature – nothing was changing. He wasn't going into withdrawal.

In just 3 weeks, John ended up walking down from 800mg of pain medication to *zero* mg. His labs improved and he was sleeping better with less pain. By simply receiving a personalized IV and botanicals, John was able to walk down from 800mg of oxycodone and never experience the debilitating effects of withdrawal.

In America we spend nearly 5 trillion on healthcare and about 75% of it goes towards chronic symptoms and illnesses like John's. Despite this effort, most chronic illnesses remain incurable. And tens of millions of Americans find themselves in similar struggles, battling their illnesses each and every day.

This struggle can cause us to lose sight that the body doesn't want to be sick either. It's ingrained in our DNA to defend ourselves, to heal ourselves, to survive. We so often look at illness as the enemy, but in sickness and in health, the body is always on your team.

Chapter 1: The Mind-Body Ecosystem

No one likes to be sick.

As we blow our nose or struggle with aching bones, we can lose sight that the body is always working really hard to help us get better.

More times than not, it does. Our noses stop running, our bones stop hurting, and we feel better.

Yet for the hundreds of millions of Americans struggling with chronic illness, their bodies aren't getting better.

Half of all adults – almost 130 million people – suffer from chronic illness(s). An estimated 50 million Americans reported issues with their mental health and nearly 50 million people are suffering from autoimmunity – where their own body is attacking and destroying itself.

The standards and reliance on medications to treat these issues has become so engrained, that it has become a problem of its own epidemic proportions where an estimated 60 million Americans are overprescribed their medications. Getting addicted to medications and other drugs is its own epidemic with up to 90% of individuals ending up back in care.

The never-ending scientific pursuit to determine how to help these diseases has illuminated a vast number of underlying factors to chronic illness and those factors can vary from person to person.

Science has shown us that there are aspects of ourselves, our environment, our culture – even the time periods we were raised in – that can all be factors in disease. It has shown that the mind can cause symptoms in our body and our body can cause symptoms in our mind. That although we tend to break the body and mind down into individual parts for study and research, it invariably functions as one whole unit.

Meet Francesca.

Fran is in her fifties and has struggled immensely with her health. She has had ruptured discs in her neck and back, breast cancer, encephalitis, Lyme disease, and neuropathy among a total of 14 chronic conditions.

As new symptoms developed over the years, new medications were added to her regimen. By the time we saw Fran, she was on a total of nine medications, three of them heavy narcotics for her constant and unbearable pain. She had been virtually immobile for the last two years.

At this point, I had spent years building upon John's story. I could never forget how peaceful he was coming off of a massive dose of oxycodone – I mean we can go without food or water longer than certain drug dependencies.

I ended up gearing my entire practice towards looking at illness from the body's perspective and helping mobilize its own natural resources. We customized a plan for Fran and spent the first two weeks of her care just supplying basic nutritional and antioxidant support.

After three weeks, Fran called her eldest brother with whom she was very close. Her voice, which had until this point been almost a whisper and conveyed a woman on the edge of death, had now regained some volume and expression.

Her brother was so shocked by the difference in Francesca's voice that he had to pull over to the side of the road for fear of bursting out in uncontrollable tears of relief. She was engaged, sharp, and laughing. She was even driving again, after being incapable of doing so for several years.

Fran called her sister-in-law who similarly broke down exclaiming. "I never thought I would hear that voice again!"

Before long, it wasn't just her voice that had changed. Her whole lively personality and mind re-emerged. Her body went from being seemingly lifeless, to dancing with her husband until the late hours of the morning.

"It's not just about a few symptoms, it's about your entire life," Fran stated. "My body is healing from the inside…and fighting and protecting me."

She was also off all of her medications.

In just a matter of weeks, her energy, sleep and cognition were now supercharged, and she was ready to tackle the world anew.

Chronic illnesses will often involve years, and in some cases, decades of your life. Francesca was weighted down with 14 different chronic ailments.

Despite it all though, she made it through. Despite multiple chronic infections and spinal fusions, and a whole heap of medications, Fran made it through.

It was like John all over again. Despite the myriad of factors that were going against her, the body still got up to move forward. It was still breathing, beating, regulating – and when it got the help it needed, it healed. The body's ingrained ability to self-heal just took over.

By this point, we were a chronic illness clinic. Symptoms ranged from chronic pain, chronic fatigue, and insomnia to chronic diseases like fibromyalgia, diabetes, and arthritis.

There were obvious differences among everyone, but there were strong similarities too. As it turns out, the body's genetic survival response is so entrenched in its DNA that it has some predictable patterns. No matter the illness, these patterns will often reveal themselves with simple standardized testing panels.

As significant as Fran presented, her biological patterns divulged themselves nonetheless,

"I don't know what to say," she said. "You saved my life."

While it is tremendously rewarding to be able to help, it is the body that does all the work. It was her body that did all the work.

Sometimes it can be hard to believe, but the role of the body doesn't change when we are sick. It will always be working to defend, to heal, to survive.

In just a couple of months, Fran went from bed bound to dancing until 2am because it's ingrained in her DNA to heal and survive. As it turns out, it's ingrained in all of our DNA to heal and survive – a pattern everybody can use to feel better.

Chapter 2: Our Cells Choices Come First

From memories, thoughts, and feelings to vital functions such as breathing, heart rate, metabolism, and more – to seamlessly defending against countless microbes, pathogens, and toxins while self-healing all the scrapes, breaks, and sickness along the way – it's hard to keep up with each and every aspect of ourselves.

Fortunately, we don't have to. The body manages much of our life for us while giving us feedback where we need to step in along the way. It doesn't guide us in Arabic or English though, but instead communicates in forms like feelings and sensations to make us more aware.

Over time we learn that when our mouths are dry, we should drink and when our stomach grumbles that we are hungry and probably should eat.

We learn when our nasal passages get stuffed up, we assume it's a sign of an allergy or a cold. Or that when a muscle hurts, we assume we have damaged it in some way. All the while, the body continues to move us forward while managing much of the day-to-day maintenance of blood pressure, metabolism, digestion, and so forth.

We are all born into a body with a predetermined set of genetic DNA. As we go through life our DNA interacts with genetic influencers, known as epigenetic factors, that turn our genes more on or off.

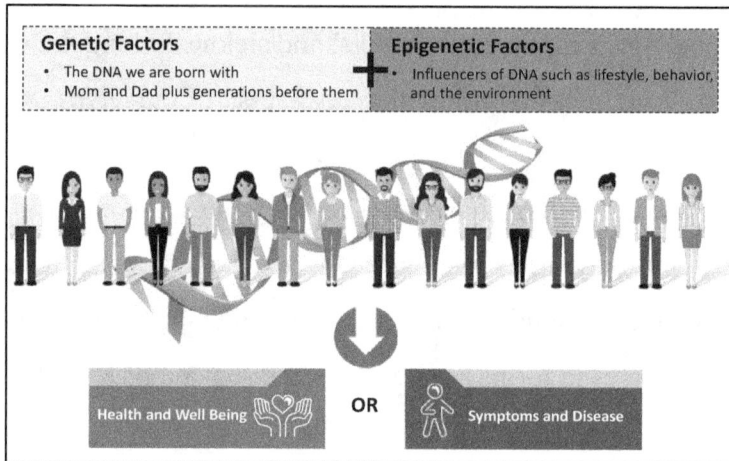

Figure 1. Factors of Health and Illness

This all happens continuously, seemingly with ease, where trillions of cells are constantly communicating with one another. We have about as many cells in our body as there are stars in our galaxy. All of these tiny little cells coming together to move larger macro systems like an orchestra playing throughout the entire mind-body.

Through billions of years of adaptive survival, our body has learned to constantly protect us while simultaneously managing the day-today, all the while adapting alongside those epigenetic influences all around us.

To give some perspective, our cells can process about *11 million bits* of information per second, compared to conscious information – the information we are aware of – that can manage about *40 bits* per second. That's about 275,000 times faster than we could possibly be aware of – for every second of every day.

Ultimately, it's impossible to be consciously aware of each and every action the body is making on our behalf; the large majority of our lives occur unconsciously and subconsciously, with little or no awareness.

The body has an entire system dedicated to continuously sensing, probing and perceiving our environment – gathering these enormous swaths of information to help the body and mind coordinate the best action on our behalf.

This system, known as the nervous system, contains over 100 billion cells that are spread everywhere throughout the brain-body. The cells, called neurons, are responsible for sensory perception – both inside and out.

They sense light, pain, smell, temperature, taste, sound, texture and more. They are the cells responsible for removing your hand from a hot stove and the ones that can move us out of the way of a moving car before we even register a conscious thought.

You can think of the nervous system as a car where the gas is known as the sympathetic nervous system, the part of the nervous system responsible for fight or flight or anything stress related. While the brakes would be the parasympathetic nervous system, the part more responsible for resting, digesting, reproduction, and healing.

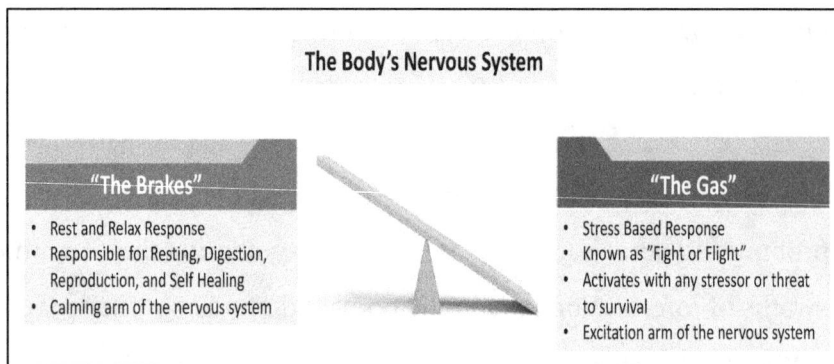

The Body's Nervous System

"The Brakes"
- Rest and Relax Response
- Responsible for Resting, Digestion, Reproduction, and Self Healing
- Calming arm of the nervous system

"The Gas"
- Stress Based Response
- Known as "Fight or Flight"
- Activates with any stressor or threat to survival
- Excitation arm of the nervous system

Figure 2. The Balance of the Nervous System

Stressors always hit the gas pedal.

Whether the stressor be mental or emotional in nature such as work, finances, or a loved one falling ill or more physical in nature like an injury or chemical imbalance – the brain-body will generate a biological response regardless. No matter the cause, there will always be an effect in the body.

This stress response is well established and contains widespread effects throughout the entire brain-body. Our heart rate increases, blood pressure and respiration increase, there is increased glucose and energy consumption, and more. The more stressful a situation is, the stronger these biological responses become.

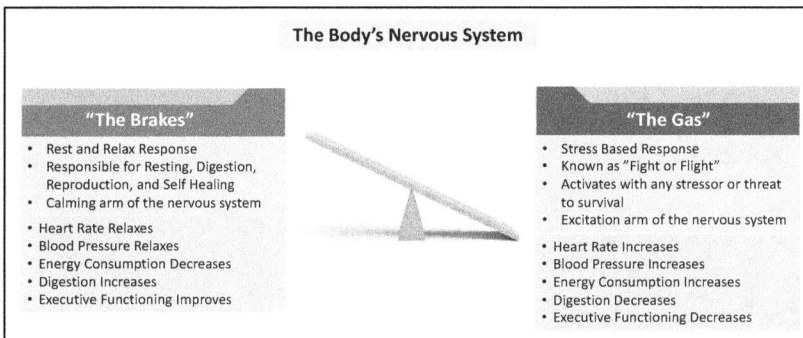

The Body's Nervous System

"The Brakes"
- Rest and Relax Response
- Responsible for Resting, Digestion, Reproduction, and Self Healing
- Calming arm of the nervous system

- Heart Rate Relaxes
- Blood Pressure Relaxes
- Energy Consumption Decreases
- Digestion Increases
- Executive Functioning Improves

"The Gas"
- Stress Based Response
- Known as "Fight or Flight"
- Activates with any stressor or threat to survival
- Excitation arm of the nervous system

- Heart Rate Increases
- Blood Pressure Increases
- Energy Consumption Increases
- Digestion Decreases
- Executive Functioning Decreases

Figure 3. Nervous System Effects on the Brain-Body

Under normal conditions, stressors often go away and these biological responses relax to balance. We get better from illness, our heartaches pass, our circumstances often change and a biofeedback loop helps shut this down and the body returns to a balanced state.

For the hundreds of millions that struggle with chronic illness, this loop stays active. Billions of neurons communicating with trillions of other cells throughout the entire brain-body for every second, for every day we struggle with a chronic condition. By the time any chronic illness is diagnosed, our cells have already made countless choices. By the time any chronic illness is diagnosed, the impact on the body can be objectively measured.

Chapter 3: Cells → Brain → Body

Getting sick is normal, getting stressed in relationships, at work, with money – it's all normal and it won't cause a chronic illness.

In fact, exercise is a form of stress. The body is built upon survival and has entire cellular systems dedicated to managing and balancing stress. Stress isn't the problem.

Chronic stress is the issue, and all chronic illnesses have resulted in some amount of chronic stress to the body – to the point where said stress is objectively evident via testing. The longer and more severe a chronic illness is, the more the entire body is involved, making this impact even more apparent.

This means that from the body's perspective, living with a chronic illness is almost as if stress never really goes away – like the gas pedal got stuck. Where any chronic illness means some amount of chronic body stress.

Chronic Illness = Chronic Body Stress

A well-coordinated effort, from our cells to the brain and ultimately throughout the entire body, this biological response is well-documented,

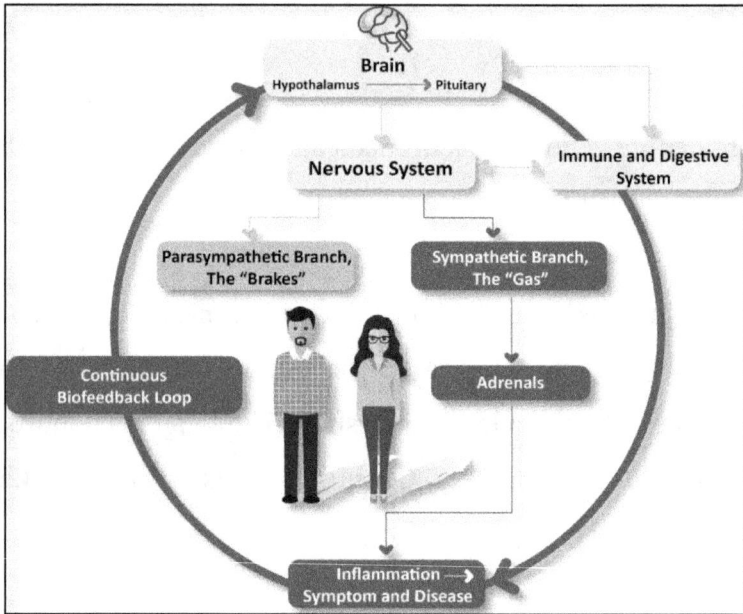

Figure 4. Chronic Stress Response: Stuck in Vicious Cycle of "Fight or Flight"

Since the brain and the nervous system are hardwired into the immune system as well as the digestive system and vice versa, all of these systems are also involved in the chronic stress response. It's one giant biofeedback loop involving trillions of cells and multiple brain-body systems – one that we are all born with.

Whether its chronic heart disease, diabetes, or addiction or chronic illnesses like anxiety, insomnia, or pain – this whole-body response will be active to some degree.

It also means that any chronic neurological illness is also an immune disorder and that chronic immune disorders have digestive and neurological components and so forth.

Over time science has continued to reinforce this multifaceted nature to chronic illness where Parkinson's, Alzheimer's, Schizophrenia, Autism, ALS and other neurological and neurodegenerative diseases are now established as autoimmune disorders.

Chronic mental health conditions, like depression and insomnia, have been noted to contribute to heart disease while heart disease has been linked with the brain as well as immune, digestive, and hormonal systems.

Nearly twenty percent of people who just think about Covid-19, get a physical symptom as a result. And more recently, multiple studies showing that a grandparent's trauma shows up in the DNA of their children and grandchildren – that this biological cascade can contribute to your illness and then be passed down to influence the DNA of your kids and their kids too.

The science has shown that it really doesn't matter where the stressor came from. That this whole-body response will be present in every chronic illness.

It has also shown that inflammation is present for every chronic illness. And that chronic stress to the body = chronic inflammation and vice versa in a sort of vicious biological feedback loop.

Ultimately, both will be present in every chronic illness – two patterns that we all share, no matter the illness.

Chronic illness = chronic body stress = chronic inflammation
Chronic illness = chronic inflammation = chronic body stress

We can work as hard as we'd like – therapies, treatments, medications – you name it – the body literally can't heal with all that inflammation and all that stress. It can't heal if it is stuck on the gas, and it can't heal without the brakes.

Treating these two genetic patterns serve as a foundation for treatment, a "step-one" for any chronic illness. Ignoring this step acts like a biological roadblock, crumbling even the most promising treatment plans.

Directly treating this genetic and biological pattern in clinical practice was most significantly expounded upon by Bessel Van der Kolk New York Time's Bestseller – *The Body Keeps the Score[1]*.

Dr. Van der Kolk described people from all walks of life some of whom underwent years of psychological and emotional therapy, yet all of their bodies were still stuck in this defensive fight or flight survival technique – even if they, themselves, had felt they had moved on from that event.

Some developed chronic mental illnesses, some struggled with pain or in relationships, some even developed autoimmune conditions – all because their bodies never let off the gas after the trauma. Tangible changes throughout the brain, mind, and body were present in each instance.

Ultimately, he helped scientifically establish that the body's perception may not be our own. That the way we see a particular life event – trauma in this case – may not be the way the body saw that event. That the body may continue to perceive stress and stay in fight or flight, even if we think we are fine. It is in fact, *"The Body [that] Keeps the Score."*

Chronic illness = chronic body stress = chronic inflammation
Chronic illness = chronic inflammation = chronic body stress

No matter how much therapy an individual does, these ingrained patterns needs to be broken, or at least dampened in order to achieve any sort of meaningful healing. It is these patterns that are our first steps that will lead to the way out.

Chapter 4: Healthcare Has a Drug Problem

Regardless of all the different established factors of chronic illness, from genetics and biochemistry to lifestyle, financials and accessibility – medications are continually expected to shoulder much of this load.

The overreliance on drugs has led to a largely silent epidemic where 1 of 6 Americans – nearly 60 million – are overprescribed their medications.

The very medications designed to treat our symptoms can often create harmful side effects, additional symptoms, and even damage our innate system. There are even studies showing that in the long term, certain medications can contribute to the very symptom or disease they are treating where opiates have been documented to cause more pain, cannabis causing irretractable nausea, and benzodiazepines contributing to anxiety and panic attacks.

You can go without food or water longer than some prescription medications where seizures and even death are labelled as side effects of withdrawal. While trying to withdrawal is an entirely separate problem altogether, where up to 90% of people seeking care for drug addiction end up back on drugs.

This epidemic only worsens as people get older where in the elderly alone,

"More than four in ten older adults take five or more prescription medications a day, an increase of 300 percent over the past two decades. Nearly 20 percent take ten drugs or more. When over-the-counter medications and supplements are included, the number of older people taking five or more drugs rises to 67 percent...

Every day, 750 older people living in the United States (age 65 and older) are hospitalized due to serious side effects from one or more medications. Over the last decade, older people sought medical treatment or visited the emergency room more than 35 million times for adverse drug events, and there were more than 2 million hospital admissions for serious adverse drug events...

Taking multiple medications also greatly increases a person's risk of suffering a serious, sometimes life-threatening side effect. Over the past few decades, medication use in the U.S., especially for older people, has gone far beyond necessary polypharmacy, to the point where millions are overloaded with too many prescriptions and are experiencing significant harm as a result."

The Lown Institute, a non-partisan think tank dedicated to transforming America's high-cost, low value health system – introduction taken from Medication Overload: America's Other Drug Problem[2]

Prescribing medications is so embedded within American society that it is to the point where millions of Americans are experiencing harm from the very medications designed to help them feel better.

"The problem of medication overload has remained hidden largely because the practice of excessive prescribing is deeply embedded in American health care. Like the air we breathe, the forces that lead to medication overload are everywhere and yet difficult to see. No single drug or class of drugs is the culprit, nor is any single disease...In most cases, no single health care professional is assigned responsibility—or has the time, training, and resources— to coordinate patient care, keep track of all the drugs patients have been prescribed, and protect them from medication overload.

Numerous forces and incentives in the U.S. health care system make it easy for clinicians to prescribe medications and difficult to scale back the dosage or deprescribe (stop a prescription). This culture of prescribing is not the fault of any one group. Health care providers, patients, and industry all play a role."[2]

We just prescribe far too many drugs.

Meet Toni.

After two bad infections within a month of one another – both requiring hospitalizations – Toni just couldn't get back on her feet. A once vibrant and outgoing teen, Toni was becoming a shell of herself. Her energy level never recovered, her joints ached every day, and her finicky stomach issues had ballooned into severe food restrictions, weight loss, and abdominal pain. Despite seeing countless doctors, no one could seem to get to the bottom of what was happening to Toni. She was now living a confined life, often not leaving the house.

When Toni arrived, she was taking the following each day:

- Tramadol 150mg (opiate like pain medication)
- Clonazepam 3mg (benzodiazepine, something like an extended release Xanax)
- Gabapentin 4000mg (antiseizure and pain medication, typical maximum dosage of 5400mg)

She started with Tramadol for pain, but then its effectiveness faded, and her doctor increased the dosage to keep up. Then more symptoms came. Then the Gabapentin was added in. Before she knew it, Toni 's health quickly got out of hand. Her symptoms and side effects were blending into one vicious cycle of health that she just couldn't escape.

If Toni walked into most doctor's offices, she would be assessed as overmedicated; however, reducing her Clonazepam alone would take nearly 2.5 years according to the widely accepted Ashton manual for benzodiazepine detox. And that treatment plan doesn't include how to manage the Clonazepam alongside Tramadol and a near max dosage of Gabapentin.

And what about why she was having pain and fatigue in the first place? Why couldn't she bounce back from that infection? Why did her stomach always seem to hurt even before the infection?

Toni received a total of 10 weeks of treatment, and she able to move away from *all* of her prescription drugs.

Her pain reduced, her brain was clear, and she was sleeping again. She had enough energy to exercise, get to the beach, and even begin some schoolwork again. Her body echoed the improvement with her laboratory values improving right alongside her symptoms. As it turned out, that infection triggered an autoimmune disease that she never knew she had and her stomach always hurt because she had celiac disease, a severe gluten intolerance. She was also significantly overprescribed.

After Toni had finished up treatment, we came to learn that Toni's home state took her driver's license because of the medications she was taking. We learned this because now, Toni is driving on her own, graduated school, working, and enjoying sports and activities again. She went on to marry and last year gave birth to a healthy baby girl.

Her mother was there on the stairwell on her last day of treatment, breaking down and exclaiming,

"You saved my daughter's life. I don't know where she'd be, where I'd be, where our family would be," she said, wiping the tears from her face.

Medications have an effective time and a place and they have saved countless lives, but we also prescribe far too many. Both can be true. I mean Prozac is now in our waterways affecting the way fish behave.

Nearly 7/10 of the 60 million overprescribed – about 42 million Americans – are on *five* or more medications, drastically increasing their chances of experiencing side effects.

Table 1: Side Effect Probability

Number of Medications	Chance of Side Effects
1	7-10%
2	14-20%
3	21-30%
4	28-40%
5	35-50%
6	42-60%
7	49-70%

*Each medication that is added, increases the chances of experiencing a side effect by 7-10%.

In America, drugs are prescribed based on the disease they are approved to treat, not for what they do to the brain and body. We use benzodiazepines for anxiety, antidepressants for depression, statins for heart disease, and so forth. Almost as if these diseases have a deficiency in pharmaceuticals – as if *we* are deficient in pharmaceuticals.

We are asking drugs to solve far too many problems and far too many factors of our illnesses. We have a drug problem. And when overserved, prescription medications become part of the illness.

Part II: Working Genetic Patterns

The body's genetic patterns are so engrained that they will physically show themselves in your body and in your labs. From a physical perspective – the body's perspective – both chronic stress and chronic inflammation will be present in each and every chronic illness.

Chronic Illness = Chronic Stress = Chronic Inflammation

More importantly, this step has to happen first for any treatment plan to be effective. Otherwise, the body remains stuck in a biological vicious cycle, unable to self-heal and unwilling to accept treatment.

Taking advantage of these ingrained patterns stops this biological cycle and begins to flip the script on your disease.

Chapter 5: Reset

The reset phase is all about hitting the brakes and laying off the gas. It is designed to address the chronic stress present in every chronic illness.

The most effective way to address this genetic pattern is by starting with those billions of tiny neurons spread throughout the entirety of the brain-body's car. This vast cellular network is like a communication highway with cells rapidly firing electrical signals to one another. This communication signal, known as a cellular action potential, is kind of like the cell's heartbeat or heart rate.

When the gas is pressed down – like in chronic illness – the cell's heart rate increases. On the other hand, the brakes help to decrease and calm down the cell's heart rate.

Our neurons' heartbeats are electrical communication signals that can be influenced faster or slower by anything that influences sensory perception. Although this is most commonly done by changing the chemical environment of the cell – like that of many pharmaceuticals – any change in pressure, temperature, chemical environments, and so forth, will all cause the cell's heart rate to fire more or less.

In fact, some of the most potent drugs affect the neurons of our car. They target either the gas or the brakes – slowing down or speeding up the cell's heartbeat.

For example, some of the most commonly used medications throughout healthcare including pain medications such as Oxycodone, Percocet, and Lyrica, among others, benzodiazepines like Xanax and Ativan, sleep aids such as Trazadone and Ambien, and even neurodegenerative drugs like Rilutek – all work by hitting the brakes and decreasing the overall heart rate of the nervous system.

Conversely, medications like steroids or amphetamines such as Adderall, Ritalin, or Vyvanse hit the gas and will increase the cell's heartbeat.

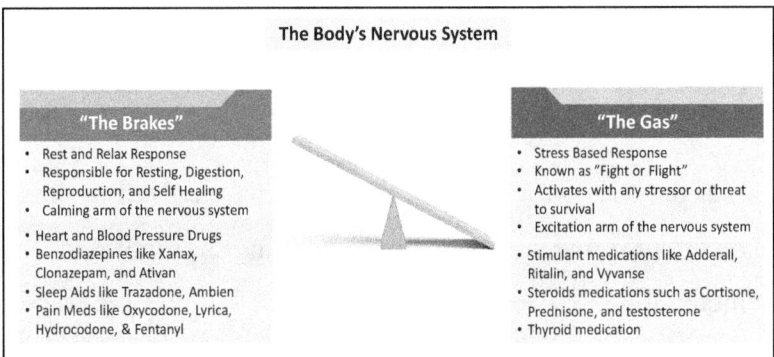

The Body's Nervous System

"The Brakes"
- Rest and Relax Response
- Responsible for Resting, Digestion, Reproduction, and Self Healing
- Calming arm of the nervous system
- Heart and Blood Pressure Drugs
- Benzodiazepines like Xanax, Clonazepam, and Ativan
- Sleep Aids like Trazadone, Ambien
- Pain Meds like Oxycodone, Lyrica, Hydrocodone, & Fentanyl

"The Gas"
- Stress Based Response
- Known as "Fight or Flight"
- Activates with any stressor or threat to survival
- Excitation arm of the nervous system
- Stimulant medications like Adderall, Ritalin, and Vyvanse
- Steroids medications such as Cortisone, Prednisone, and testosterone
- Thyroid medication

Figure 5. Drugs and the Nervous System

Many nutraceuticals such as theanine, 5-htp, and magnesium decrease the cell's heart rate too, along with botanicals like valerian root, chamomile, and passionflower.

Although the administration, timing, and dosages of these various chemicals can be unique per person, per illness, every chronic illness needs them in some way shape or form. Every chronic illness has hit the gas too much and every chronic illness needs more brakes.

Meet Sharon. Sharon is 45 and has a history of 15 chronic disorder diagnoses ranging from fibromyalgia, brain fog, and kidney disease to complex regional pain syndrome, migraines, and asthma.

"I've had a total of 29 procedures or hospitalizations and I've seen at least 14 different doctors," she exclaimed when arriving at our clinic.

"I feel like I have been sick as long as I can remember."

Sharon was on a total of 17 different medications including two different opiates for pain, one being a high dose of 150 mg methadone.

There is no question her body and mind have taken some stress over the years – some of which occurred well before she had the ability to take her first steps.

"I'll do whatever you tell me to do. I need to feel better for my son, he's only 8 – I feel like he's only ever seen me sick."

To best serve her, many different treatments and therapies would need to be employed. Sharon would have to make changes too. But first, we had to hit the brakes. We had to reset her cell's heartbeat.

From the significant stress and medication overload of all of her illnesses, her body was stuck on the gas pedal and hadn't used the brakes for years. Sharon had already tried countless psychotherapies, undergone numerous surgeries, drug interventions, sound therapies, meditations, and so much more. Yet no matter the mental effort, medication or lifestyle changes, no matter what she did or how hard she seemed to try, her body remained stuck in a vicious biological state of fight or fight, unable to overcome the physical burden of the disease – unable to improve.

As with John, Fran, and Toni, we utilized a blend of botanicals and natural IV compounds to help Sharon's body hit the brakes and lay off the gas. Treating this underlying factor works to allow the body to biologically relax, directly improving symptoms and the efficacy of any concurrent or subsequent therapies.

By this time, I had been working towards proprietary formulations that were largely geared towards both causes of all chronic illness – reducing inflammation and this chronic stress response. We had administered tens of thousands of IVs and every IV had chemicals to hit the brakes and antioxidants to reduce inflammation. The labs, symptoms, and any medications would determine how much of each to use and for how long.

After four weeks of our IV therapy at four times per week, Sharon's pain and balance were improved to the point that she no longer needed her cane. For the first time in two years, she was able to walk completely on her own.

After six weeks, her brain fog began to clear while her labs values reflected her significant improvement. After a total of eight weeks of therapy, Sharon was able to reduce her medication load from seventeen medications to nine, not only eliminating both of her pain medications entirely but also six additional overprescribed medications.

Sharon's liver enzymes also normalized, her glucose levels were no longer prediabetic, and Sharon's CV risk, her risk of having a cardiovascular event like a stroke or heart attack, went from high to low (CRP 11.1 to 1.7).

After decades of decline, Sharon was like a new person. She had energy, less pain, and her brain was clear. Sharon felt renewed, with quite the pep in her step. Maybe even too much pep in fact.

"Mom you may need to tone it down a bit," her son said to her during her follow-up visit.

"I have to make up for all that lost time," she told him. "Trust me," he said to her, "You are."

Chapter 6: Restore

All chronic illnesses have well documented inflammation. This inflammation can be unique to the disease as well as a result of the chronic stress response. But it will always be there.

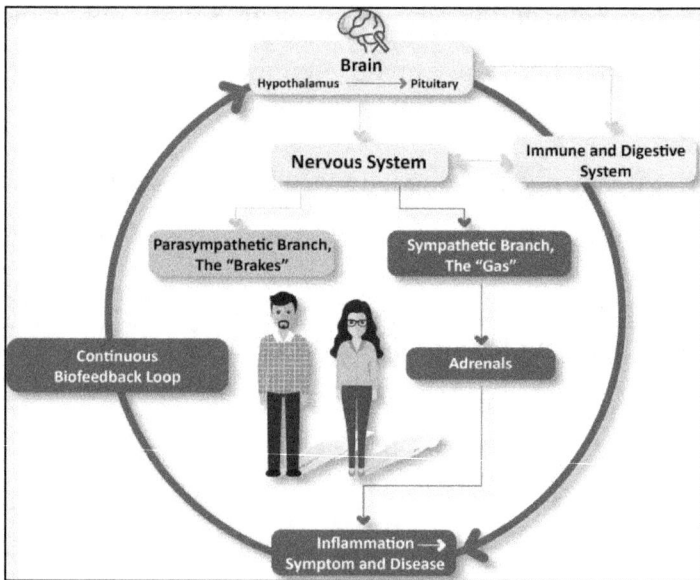

Figure 4. Chronic Stress Response

By the time chronic illness is diagnosed, both chronic stress and chronic inflammation are now a continuous whole-body cycle. Each aspect of this cycle has been activated an innumerable amount of times. The cells may be the leader in illness, but as you can see from Figure 4, many aspects of the brain-body have been impacted by the chronic illness.

The Restore phase is about reducing any noted inflammatory impacts of the illness. This includes inflammation as a result of the chronic stress response seen in Figure 4. Both of these underlying causes of chronic illness come with reliable lab values that can literally gauge the impact that the chronic illness has had on the body.

Table 2: Testable Lab Values

Area of the Brain-Body	Testable Labs
Brain (Pituitary Hormones)	*ACTH, ADH, TSH, Prolactin, FSH, LH*
Adrenal Glands	*Cortisol, DHEA*
Immune System	*WBC, CD4/CD8*
Digestive System	*WBC, CMP, Ferritin*
Other Hormones	*Free T3, Testosterone, Estrogen, Progesterone*
Inflammatory Markers	*CRP, HbA1c, TGFb, C4a, C3a, MMP-9, Ferritin*

Labs are like helping the body talk to us in a universal standardized language. It's like revealing which areas of the body need to be improved in order to help us feel better. You need to run enough tests to provide enough context to these ingrained pathways, to provide enough context of the illness from the body's perspective.

Conversely, this isn't an exhaustive list; it is meant to frame the body in terms of chronic stress and inflammation – the two biological factors present in every chronic illness.

As with the Reset Phase, IV therapy is the backbone for the Restore Phase providing several antioxidants alongside calming brake chemistry. Oral antioxidants are used too, helping to reinforce a successful Reset and Restoration.

Inflammation though, like stressors, can come from a wide variety of sources. This means that antioxidants and antidotes can too. You'd be surprised at how additional antidotes like dietary changes, balancing stressful work environments, and ditching toxic relationships can literally shape your DNA, especially after these two biological roadblocks are removed.

Part III: Shaping Your Own DNA

Chronic illness involves all of our DNA. From ingrained biological pathways to our emotions, lifestyle, relationships, and environments – by the time a chronic illness is diagnosed, it has all blended together.

We are all capable of influencing our DNA. Our lifestyle, behavior, and our environment – these universal aspects of our lives – literally shape our DNA. And ultimately it is up to us whether that influence is positive or negative.

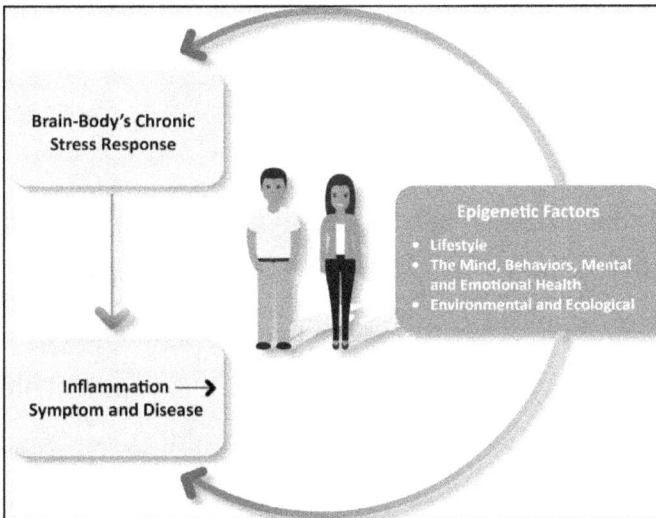

Figure 6. Other Influencing Factors of Stress of Inflammation

While Reset and Restore work within the body's engrained patterns of illness, there are also aspects of our DNA that can be flipped on or off by epigenetic factors – influencers of DNA that are more in our control.

Once these biological roadblocks are removed, it is time to turn to the most significant influencers of DNA:
Lifestyle (Chapter 7),
Behavior (Chapters 8 and 9), and the
Environment (Chapter 10)

Your day-to-day lifestyle includes core needs of the body such as what we eat and drink every day, while behaviors can be anything from beliefs we hold to how we act in close relationships. Our environment is our surroundings.

This also means this phase in healing can be a continuous work in progress. It involves where you live, the relationships you keep, it involves looking at yourself, making changes, considering how life events have affected you, and looking at the countless other factors that have been proven to impact your health. Most importantly, it involves ensuring these known influencers of our DNA are helping us get better, not keeping us sick.

Chapter 7: Start with Lifestyle

Lifestyle is essentially a long-term investment in your health. You may get lucky, win the lottery and feel better right away, but for most of us – the effect is slowly built over time.

The reverse is true too. Eating a bag of chips isn't going to get you chronically sick. The same is true if you stop exercising for a bit or have a stressful period at work or in a relationship.

This influencer of DNA is the sum of our choices – day in and day out – that can ultimately contribute to your illness or help heal it.

While this means the effects or changes to lifestyle aren't felt overnight and require consistency, it also creates a path where everyday necessities for the body, like eating, drinking, and moving, provide daily opportunities to create a positive influence on our DNA. It's like a daily opportunity for your lifestyle to serve as medicine.

Food and Water

As development of the earth continues, farming has evolved into an industry that has become increasingly efficient at maximizing production. Different chemicals and pesticides are so widely used –

an estimated 1 billion pounds per year in the US alone – that they are now a part of our food and water supply. And by the time our food is picked, packed, transported, and unpacked for our shelves, it can lose up to 90% of its vital nutrients (not including the time the food spends in your fridge!).

Processed foods have even more chemicals, crazy high salt, and even less nutrients. For "food to be thy medicine," start out by eating less out of wrappers and more out of your fridge. If one thing is for certain, eating more processed and less whole foods has consistently been shown to decrease life span as well as contribute to mental illness and chronic diseases including cancer, diabetes, and autoimmunity.

If you have severe symptoms or diseases affecting your brain, immune or digestive system – you should avoid additional inflammatory foods like dairy and gluten while working to incorporate more antioxidants, such as berries, into your diet.

Otherwise, you don't need to go too crazy over it. Eat whole foods, cook most of your meals, don't eat too many processed and fast foods. You'd be surprised at how this simple change can make you feel.

Do the same for what you are drinking too. Avoid sugary drinks and opt for water – some sort of filtered water. Our tap water and fresh water streams, like that of our crop and livestock supply, is now integrated with different chemicals and pesticides and require filtration.

Contaminants like forever chemicals, a group of chemicals that take "forever" (a really long time) to break down and go away, have now been found present in 70% of rivers worldwide with 26 million Americans being exposed to toxic limits of this chemical. Our oceans, lakes, and rivers are infested with them where it's literally raining forever chemicals in Miami and probably everywhere else too. This contamination has percolated its way into fish, animals, and people across the U.S., where they have been consistently documented to cause cancer, reproductive issues, and autoimmunity among other serious health issues (watch the movie *Dark Waters* for an overview and powerful true story about forever chemicals).

Plastics, pesticides, contaminants, and many other industrial and environment toxins have been linked with deadly and debilitating disease where most of us are exposed to them in little quantities over time. This often makes it difficult to see cause and effect. Eating that cheeseburger won't kill you, and neither will ingesting a few chemicals here and there. But consistently eating processed foods or drinking contaminated water is like death by a thousand cuts – slowly but surely pushing your body towards illness. We can limit our exposure to these known health hazards and positively influence our own DNA by simply eating more whole foods, drinking filtered water, and avoiding chemicals and plastics wherever possible.

Movement

From the largest of stars and the tiniest of particles to trillions of our very own cells firing trillions of times every moment – movement is a fundamental feature throughout the entire universe.

The less you move, the worse you'll likely feel. Decreased exercise has been linked with autoimmunity, memory issues, decreased life span, as well as a slew of mental illness symptoms. Conversely exercise has been shown to increase mood, decrease anxiety, protect the heart, increase life span, and more.

Despite these well-known positive effects of movement and exercise, the symptoms of chronic illness often make it difficult to get healthy movement in. If it's your first time back, start slowly, and pick something easy or something you know you will keep up with. Light walks or a few balance or weight bearing exercises are a great starting point. Get some help if you need it. It really doesn't matter what you do, you just have to move. If you can move enough to sweat, even better.

Go Outside

As if they are stopping for a coffee on a break, many Japanese and Koreans are paying just to sit and stare at nature. In many European countries, national parks are prescribed as therapy where getting into nature in any regard is so effective for your health, it can be reimbursed under insurance. Just touching the earth with your body, known as grounding, has been shown to help with pain, improve immunity, and even decrease inflammation.

It doesn't have to be long and you don't even have to do something – just get yourself outside for a bit. Breathe some fresh air, feel the warmth of the sun, touch the ground, plan an adventure – the body needs it all every day. As a species, we've spent the last few hundred thousand years completely in nature where today the National Institute of Health estimates we spend up to 90% of our time indoors. Go outside.

Breathe

Just Breathe.

In *One Nation Under Stress,* Dr. Sanjay Gupta, shows that for the first time in our nation's history, the life expectancy went down. We are dying earlier, despite spending trillions each year on healthcare. And we are more stressed than ever[3].

Breathing is one of the first areas to be affected when we get stressed and is one of the only automatic involuntary actions we have some control over. As outstandingly outlined in James Nestor's New York Times Best Seller, *Breath,* we take 20,000 breaths per day extracting oxygen as our primary energy source – doing it efficiently can go a long way[4].

Since it is well established the body is under chronic stress by definition of a chronic illness, it is vitally important we control the stressors we are able to.

Stressors come in all shapes and sizes from work, finances, and relationships, to basic needs, shelter and safety. Identify all that you can, even if there's nothing you can do about it. If you don't know where to start – just slow down and breathe.

Your Lifestyle, Your Influence

All of these aspects of your lifestyle influence your DNA. Each choice gives you the opportunity to change the way you feel – to have more power and control of your illness.

More recently, Dr. Rhonda Patrick went on to speak in front of the Senate Aging Commission and outlined our reality in America and how necessary these lifestyle aspects are for our DNA, for our health and well-being.

"If you want to meaningfully impact aging in America, start with obesity—few things erode longevity and quality of life as profoundly, accelerating the biological aging process and fueling nearly every major chronic disease. Obesity alone is linked to 13 types of cancer and cuts life expectancy by 3–10 years, depending on severity. It promotes DNA damage and accelerates our fundamental aging process—often measured by epigenetic age. It's one of the principal differences between the U.S. and many of the world's longest-lived nations.

We're overfed but undernourished. 60% of all calories Americans consume come from ultra-processed foods that:

- Fail to induce proper satiety, pushing us to overeat.

- Remain cheaper than whole foods, economically incentivizing the least healthy choices
- Hijack our dopamine reward pathways, reinforcing addictive eating behaviors.

This trifecta—no satiety, low cost, and built-in addictiveness—keeps us in a cycle of poor health outcomes and runaway healthcare costs.

But caloric excess is only part of the problem—we are also nutrient-deficient. Low omega-3 levels—affecting 80 to 90% of Americans—carry the same mortality risk as smoking. Vitamin D deficiency—easily corrected—compromises immune function, cognition, and longevity. Nearly half of Americans don't get enough magnesium—impairing DNA repair and increasing the risk of cancer.

We are not solving these problems—we are medicating them. The average American over 65 takes five or more prescription drugs daily—stacking interactions that compound in unpredictable ways. We must start treating physical inactivity as a disease. It carries the same mortality risk as smoking, heart disease, and diabetes. Going from a low cardiorespiratory fitness to a low normal adds 2.1 years to life expectancy. By age 50, many Americans have already lost

10% of their peak muscle mass. By 70, many have lost up to 40%. This isn't just about looking strong. It's about survival.

- Higher muscle mass means improved insulin sensitivity - it means a 30% lower mortality risk.
- Grip strength is a stronger predictor of cardiovascular mortality - the number one cause of death in the United States - than high blood pressure
- The strongest middle-aged adults have a 42% lower dementia risk.

And yet, we treat resistance training as optional. It is not. It is the most powerful intervention we have against aging including increasing muscle mass, strength and bone density. Hip fractures alone kill 20–60% of older adults within a year. This is a death sentence we can prevent with resistance training - which has been shown to lower fracture risk by 30-40%. The current RDA for protein is too low for older adults. Studies have shown when it's increased by half this reduces frailty by 32%, while doubling it, combined with resistance training, increases muscle mass by 27% and strength by 10% more than training alone. If we want to prevent muscle loss and frailty, we must update our protein recommendations and prioritize strength training.

We must foster a culture of American exceptionalism built on daily, effortful exercise. Not as an afterthought. Not as a luxury. But as a non-negotiable foundation for aging, but also clear thinking, resilience, and even leadership. The body and brain are not separate. The consequences of poorly regulated blood sugar, sedentary living, and muscle loss are not just physical—they affect cognition, judgment, and resilience. We cannot medicate our way out of what we have behaved our way into." *Dr. Rhonda Patrick, Senate Aging Commission*[5].

In Japan, they went insofar to make lifestyle the law, where "in 2002, Japan took the remarkable action of stipulating by law that citizens must deepen their interest in and understanding of the importance of healthy lifestyle habits, be aware of their own health status, and strive to improve their health throughout their lives."[6]

There is no question that lifestyle is medicine. Even in our own country, in the late 70s, Dr. Dean Ornish went insofar as to claim he would reverse heart disease with lifestyle alone, and he did. Some years later, his program is covered by insurance for the effectiveness of his lifestyle therapy in stopping and reversing heart disease, the number one chronic illness killing the most Americans. One genetic influencer – lifestyle – has been shown to cure heart disease on its own.

The science will only continue to cement how significant lifestyle is for your illness and ultimately your health. In the end, the choices we make surrounding lifestyle are daily choices that can either serve as medicine or slowly poison us by a thousand cuts.

Chapter 8: Mindset

"I don't think I can do that," Brian stated, seemingly unsure of himself.

"You can't or you won't?" his doctor replied to him.

Brian sat there for a moment as he thought about the doctor's response. It had been years since he had walked on his own without his wheelchair.

The recovery from his surgery was supposed to be 8 weeks. Multiple surgeries and an unfortunate accident turned 8 weeks into *four years*. Brian never imagined he'd even be in this position. He was only 31 years old.

"Your neurologist is right, you'll probably be in pain," the doctor said to him. "But it's less pain than when you started. And your energy level is drastically improved."

After just three weeks of therapy, his pain was coming down and his brain was sharp, gaining clarity with each treatment. As his symptoms improved so did his testing, but it also revealed he would likely always have some level of pain and long-term neuropathy.

When it comes to chronic illness, the mind doesn't just sit on the sidelines. The mind and body work in unison like a live action ecosystem. Where the body goes so does the mind and vice versa. In sickness and in health, the body and mind go hand in hand.

> *Chronic illness = chronic body stress = chronic mind stress*
> *Chronic illness = chronic mind stress = chronic body stress.*

You don't have to answer the chicken (mind) or the egg (body) when it comes to chronic illness; it's both at this point. Whether the body initially caused the symptoms in the mind or vice versa, by the time a chronic illness is diagnosed – both are always involved.

Any memory that is formed and stored in our DNA comes from a mashup up from both the body and the mind of all the sensations, emotions, and thoughts around a given event or circumstance. The more that memory promotes or threatens survival, the stronger the positive or negative influence is on our DNA.

> A Memory =
> thoughts from the mind + feelings and sensations + however we perceive it

Brian had the physical trauma from the surgery and the emotional trauma from it going wrong and him ultimately not recovering all these years later. At this point, his emotions, sensations, pains, and thoughts were all blending into the collective memory of the trauma. It was a strong memory for him.

As his brain-body began to physically heal from all that trauma, it was time to move to the effect his pain and surgeries have had on his mental health, too. He began to realize how some of his thoughts, constructs, and beliefs have formed around his illness. That he was tired, foggy, and in pain but he was also unhappier, scared, and hopeless, too.

"It's not your fault that you are sick," doctor began. "No one is blaming you that you were in an accident, that you needed these surgeries – I'd be significantly affected by that too, anyone would. But you have to address that affect, it's still your responsibility to try and change that, if you can."

I never forgot that conversation. No matter what has happened to you, no matter the disease, you aren't to blame or at fault – but you are responsible. In the end, it still falls on you to have a mindset that helps you heal.

As with lifestyle, the state our mind is now well established to either contribute to illness or help heal it. In other words – you can create a healthier body by having a healthier mind, just as your mind will feel better with a healthier body. Sometimes this can mean being more positive, and sometimes it means reworking entire attitudes and patterns surrounding your health and illness. Regardless, these aspects of ourselves are undoubtedly affected by our illnesses, a factor that we can all do more to address.

It is estimated that 20% of adults, or 50 million Americans, struggle with their mental health. Another estimated 15 million children have a mental health disorder with only 2/10 getting the treatment they need.

Moreover, the individuals that receive therapy are often from chronic mental illnesses such as anxiety, depression, and mood disorders while the mental effect of chronic diseases like fibromyalgia, heart disease, and diabetes often goes overlooked.

Any effective treatment plan will incorporate your mental and emotional health – merely as a result of having a chronic illness. To me, therapy is simply acknowledging that the mind can have a role in your illness and that it has been impacted from being sick every day. It's acknowledging that you were affected by your illness and that maybe there are ways you could learn to understand it better, handle it better, even feel better.

You aren't admitting fault or blame for causing your illness by accepting the help you need, nor does it always have a large impact for every illness.

But it always has an impact. Our mind is invariably impacted by chronic illness – just as the body is. And our perspective, our beliefs, our behaviors – they all matter. All of it can fundamentally influence our DNA and impact how we feel.

We ultimately got Brian the help he needed and integrated it alongside the necessary physical therapies and treatments to get him better.

And after four weeks of IVs and six more weeks of working hard with physical and emotional therapists, Brian began walking again and never looked back. He's been entirely without his wheelchair for the last seven years.

Chapter 9: Explore Behavior and its Beginnings

Just as the body has predetermined patterns that exist from birth, the mind does too. From the moment we are born, these patterns are shaping our behaviors and our DNA.

As some of the underlying factors and core needs of the body are being healed, the mind will begin to heal too. But if its behaviors, constructs, and patterns surrounding illness, do not – eventually the body will be pulled back down into the illness.

It's hard to imagine that how we act and how we go about our relationships can fundamentally shape our DNA. That our behavior can literally keep us healthy or make us sick; some of which is shaped well before we even have conscious agency. There's a difference between being aware of something and having control over it.

From the moment we are born, many different behaviors, relationships, and beliefs are already being formed much before we are aware of them. This means that the foundation of our behavior has already been laid down before we ever got sick.

Some of the most significant impacts on our behavior as adults stem from two crucial biological processes of our upbringing, known as attachment and attunement.

Broadly speaking, they are exactly as they sound. As we can't take care of ourselves as young infants and children, we *attach* to whoever is around and *tune into* how they solve problems and work with others – how they make it in the world we were just born into.

Attachment and attunement will occur with whomever are the primary caregivers, typically our parents. And both of these processes – through any upbringing – will create lasting influences on the body and mind and ultimately our health.

Attachment was initially framed by British psychoanalyst John Bowlby, who had experiences working with traumatized and children separated from their parents during the course of World War II.

Bowlby posited that the relationships with caregivers during the first eighteen months of life were critical in laying down the foundations of one's relationship with others as well as self-concept.

Different circumstances and upbringings promote different attachment styles, and the impact of attachment will manifest in many ways throughout life, influencing all social relationships and especially intimate ones.

For example, people with avoidant attachment styles, tend to be very withdrawn and don't disclose much of themselves. While people with anxious attachment will be very concerned about the stability of their relationships and be constantly worrying about abandonment.

All attachment styles blend with how our dependent caregivers teach us how to react to other people and life's circumstances. This second process, known as attunement, forms the basis of empathy and compassion, or lack thereof.

Dr. Dan Siegel, clinical professor of psychology at UCLA, says, "Children need attunement to feel secure and to develop well, and throughout our lives we need attunement to feel close and connected." Our kids need to see how we solve problems, care for them and for others, and manage the world we live in.

Parents and significant others often serve as our sole models of connection in early life and will ingrain both of these fundamental patterns within our life. They also shoulder much of the responsibility for the amount of exposure to stress and dangerous situations growing up.

They have the responsibility not to traumatize us directly or expose us to overly stressful situations, but also shield us from the any trauma in our environment and the world around us, despite those circumstances often being out of their control. They have the responsibility, regardless of the circumstances, to ingrain healthy attachment and attunement processes – to ingrain healthy influences on our DNA.

I remember just two years ago when my wife and I were trekking through our own water-soaked clothes and furniture after hurricane Ian destroyed what used to be our home for the last seven years, and wondering how different it would be if we had our son with us. I couldn't imagine also being responsible for appropriately shielding my son from stripping every bit of our home to the studs, losing our cars, and tossing nearly everything we had to the curb that now piled nearly fifteen feet high, full of appliances, floorings, dry wall, furniture, and anything we owned. I just remember thinking how it would have affected him. Will it affect how we raise him, where we will raise him? How has it affected us?

Early environmental stress and developmental trauma caused by things like toxic caregiving, natural disasters, parental separation, war and other traumatic events have enduring effects on the nervous system and regulation of the body's chronic stress response.

Prolonged separation or permanent separation/object loss has been associated with dysregulation of the chronic stress response later in life, leaving the mind-body exposed to a known underlying risk factor of all chronic illness. Exposure to enough stress can shape the largest of neurons and even kill them.

Exposure to trauma and these types of highly stressful circumstances during upbringing has also been shown to have lasting impacts on emotional regulation, our memory systems as well as previously mentioned areas of the brain including the hypothalamus, pituitary, hippocampus, and the limbic center, among others.

The effects are so prominent and well documented that Dr. Van der Kolk in *The Body Keeps the Score* went so far as to say that any patient that is positive for autoimmunity should be checked for childhood trauma. That a body-based disease as an adult has roots in behaviors that were shaped as a child.

There is even evidence that separation from a caregiver in the context of family discord (including mother–infant attachment-bond disruption) may have greater effects than even the actual death of a parent.

Our caregivers have significant and lasting impacts on our DNA and ultimately our health and well-being. By the time a chronic illness is diagnosed, it can be hard to see how the way we were raised may be contributing to the chronic illness we are experiencing today – some decades later. The effect of our upbringing can seem so distant from our illness that much of the time, we often remain unaware of its undeniable impact.

While not everyone will have their upbringing fundamental to their chronic illness, everyone's DNA is shaped by their own behavior and their own upbringing. Eighty percent of brain development and how your child goes about speech, language, thinking, social relationships, and more is already formed by age three. Ninety percent is formed by age five.

Do you like who you are, how you act, how you treat yourself?

How do you treat your loved ones, your parents?

Do they make you a better person?

It's up to you whether you like the answers, and it's up to you to change them if you don't. If you can't change them on your own, there is help.

Your behavior towards yourself and your behavior within relationships will always have an impact on your health. Poor behavior and toxic relationships are breeding grounds for chronic illness. Poor behavior and toxic relationships that began from childhood are often underlying factors for chronic illness.

More importantly, caring for yourself and doing what is right by your body, your mind, and your loved ones literally does just the opposite; it makes you stronger, it helps improve chronic illness, and it invests in healthy DNA for yourself and your kids' future.

Part IV: Getting Better

Just as there is no one cause for chronic illness, there is no one way to get better. There are also no magic formulas laying around that somehow everyone with chronic illness seemed to miss. The science continues to show that there are a multitude of causes for each chronic illness, and that those causes can vary from person to person. The science also continues to show that you can get better too. That you can cure your quality of life without ever curing your disease.

Chapter 10: Build Your Own Pharmhouse

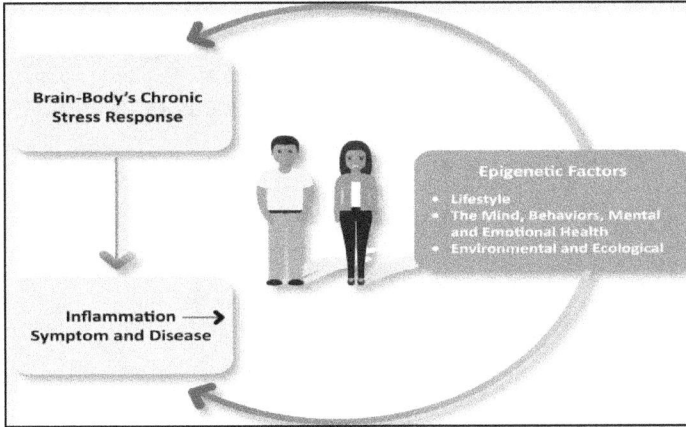

Figure 6. Other Influencing Factors of Stress of Inflammation

It is next to impossible to sustain progress without a healthy environment. From the air you breathe to the amount of trees in your neighborhood to the stability of your home and government, staying better depends on the health of your environment and ecology.

A few years ago, I expanded our indoor clinic to include a 1-acre outdoor space. The property helps to bridge the gap between all of the learning and treatment at our medical clinic and the necessary integration it takes when you return home. It acts sort of like a mini community where people could practice what it was like to feel better and learn what it would take to stay better in their own environments. To learn what it would take to ensure their environments are helping them get better, not keeping them sick.

There are therapies like acupuncture, meditation, massage, saunas, cold pools, talks, and games, as well as occasional events that often include art therapy, cooking, and animal-assisted therapy – all taking place throughout the lush tropical space.

People move from activity to activity receiving treatment from different providers, talking in groups, and working out their own treatment plans. After everyone has had the opportunity to move through all of the different therapies and exercises, we all gather to eat a light lunch. It's like an adult day camp for rehabbing chronic illnesses – we call it the pharmhouse.

Patients are able to participate in both individual and group therapy, while their loved ones – often the silent warriors of chronic illnesses – are encouraged to join in. Everyone is able to ask questions to the very doctors and practitioners providing their care. In real time, patients can work to understand and implement their treatment plans right alongside other patients, family members, and their medical team.

It has helped individuals come a long way in their recovery. From social interactions and lifestyle skills to getting out of your head and trying new therapies, the pharmhouse is a place for patients to be supported by an entire community – nature included.

We spend the necessary time inside the clinic working through medical histories, going through labs, administering various therapies – including the IVs – and the outside space allowed them the experience of maintaining all of this in a real-world environment. It's the best of both worlds.

All of science agrees that lifestyle, behavior, and environment are the three most significant influencers of DNA, yet treatment plans rarely address these factors for illness. You can do simple things like get an air purifier to help the health of your environment – and you should – but I really wanted to teach people how to turn their living environments into a healing ecosystem that would ensure they stayed better.

I ended up finding a way to turn the environment into a real and reproducible therapy for our patients and teach them how to implement this alongside their loved ones and outside of a medical setting – in their everyday life setting. This was a space we could teach and reinforce these concepts, but quite literally provide that healthy environment for the DNA to heal. Individual progress went faster, farther, and maintained better than it ever had before.

The idea for the pharmhouse stemmed from work done by psychologist, Abraham Maslow (of the hierarchy of needs) who outlined that while we all have highly stressful, sometimes traumatic experiences that occur throughout our life, *we also have really awesome peak experiences too.*

Like that of trauma and other stressful or dangerous events in our past, the body strongly associates all the components that went into that particular event. It does the same with good feelings and good events, too – ones that help us move forward and provide us with support, love, curiosity, freedom, and more.

Whether it's a particular event like the birth of a child or getting your dream job or an important place or person like the mountains or a loved one, we can call upon peak experiences and relevant purposes in our life to help us get better.

Time seemingly disappears where the body and mind can be transported directly back into those experiences, especially if they have had a significant impact on our life – whether positive or negative. While triggers transport us to negative experiences, we can surround ourselves with facilitators that can continually transport us to peak experiences – to some of the best feelings we've ever had.

Not only does this help people feel better, but it allows for the body and mind to associate intense feelings and thoughts with something more positive, instead of associating it with feeling poorly all the time or triggering the stresses from our past.

Start to immerse yourself with everything that will help your progress and remove the things that will hinder it. Start to incorporate as many things, people, places, senses, and therapies that reinforce these feelings – that help you feel the way you want to feel. Whether it be a room in your house, a holistic team of doctors, a cold tank outside amongst nature and friends – or all of the above – build out whatever your own community looks like for you. That's the environment your DNA needs to get better, to stay better.

Just like there are sights, sounds, feelings, and memories that will trigger the body into a traumatic state, these same sensations and memories can also facilitate a pretty awesome peak experience too. Our senses are involved in so much more than we realize. To the point where improving body awareness can improve motor neuron diseases like Parkinson's and improving senses like smell, hearing, and sight have all been shown to reduce symptoms of dementia.

Instead of working to delete all of the negative associations we have with difficult events in our life, we can work to replace these associations with different experiences – with positive and peak ones. From the simplest of senses to our most intimate relationships and core needs, we don't exist separate from our surroundings. Real life doesn't take place with your doctor or in a room with four walls with your therapist talking about what it's like to get better. It occurs with people, with places, with the environment. And it's continuously occurring.

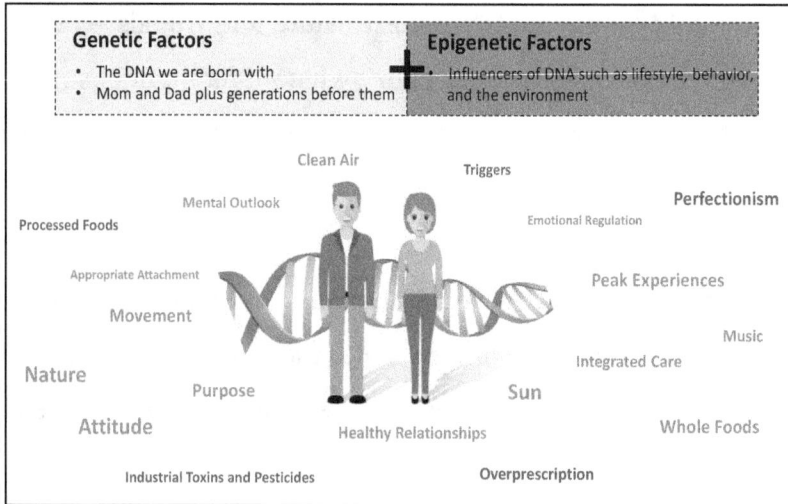

Figure 7. Creating your own Community

The body pulls the mind which can pull the body and vice versa, which can all be pulled by our environment. Building you own community – creating your own pharmhouse – ensures you DNA is being pulled in a healthy direction.

Chapter 11: Putting it all Together

Most chronic illnesses remain incurable with many different underlying causes ranging from genetic factors, ones that are predetermined – to epigenetic factors, genetic influencers like lifestyle, behaviors, and the environment.

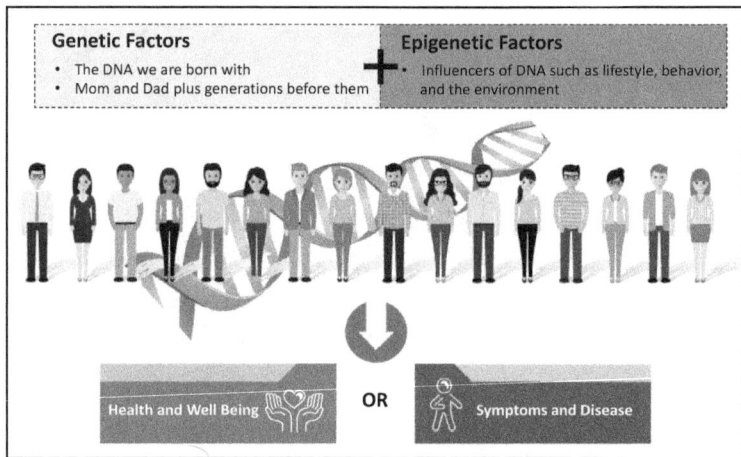

Figure 1. Factors of Health and Illness

Despite our perspective of taking, loss, struggle and illness, the body is merely a signal that something is off, that it needs some help

The body is always looking out for you. It has taken billions of years to get to this point and it's designed to defend, to heal, to survive. Its role doesn't change when we are sick despite how the illness makes us feel. It's still trying to help you and is forever on your team. (Chapter 1).

Our cells choices far outnumber our own (275,000 to 1 – every second of every day) and ultimately lead the way – long before disease is diagnosed. By the time this occurs, tangible stress has already occurred to the body and mind. Too much gas and not enough brakes is a biological underlying cause in all chronic illness. It's such an ingrained genetic pathway that it reveals itself through testing (Chapter 3).

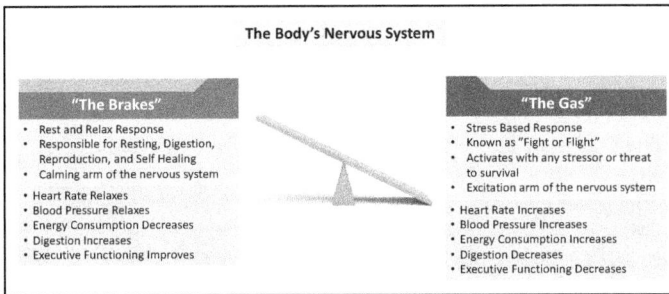

The Body's Nervous System

"The Brakes"
- Rest and Relax Response
- Responsible for Resting, Digestion, Reproduction, and Self Healing
- Calming arm of the nervous system
- Heart Rate Relaxes
- Blood Pressure Relaxes
- Energy Consumption Decreases
- Digestion Increases
- Executive Functioning Improves

"The Gas"
- Stress Based Response
- Known as "Fight or Flight"
- Activates with any stressor or threat to survival
- Excitation arm of the nervous system
- Heart Rate Increases
- Blood Pressure Increases
- Energy Consumption Increases
- Digestion Decreases
- Executive Functioning Decreases

Figure 3. Nervous System Effects on the Brain-Body

Chronic illness = chronic stress to the body, and as the cells→brain→body, the chronic stress response becomes a whole-body response. This inflammation, in addition to the inflammation that occurs throughout the brain-body in any chronic illness, is another biological underlying cause of all chronic illnesses and also measurable via testing.

> *Chronic illness = chronic body stress = chronic inflammation*
> *Chronic illness = chronic inflammation = chronic body stress*

By the very scientific nature of chronic illness, both the body and mind are involved, where ultimately every neurological condition is also an immune and digestive one and vice versa.

> *Chronic Illness = chronic neuro = chronic immune = chronic digestive*

Help for our illnesses often comes by way of medications, where these drugs are expected to solve multiple genetic and epigenetic factors of our illness – all in one pill. This overreliance on prescription medications has led to a largely silent epidemic with nearly 60 million overprescribed their medications (Chapter 4).

This can all make it difficult to know where to start with a treatment plan, let alone getting better. Start by reflecting the two underlying factors of all chronic illness. Start with the body first. Reduce your stress response and get your brain and body physically calmed down (Chapter 5). Reduce your inflammation (Chapter 6).

As your brain-body is being supported through a good Reset and Restoration, focusing on the factors that are more in your control adds viable therapies, improves quality of life, and literally helps improve your DNA.

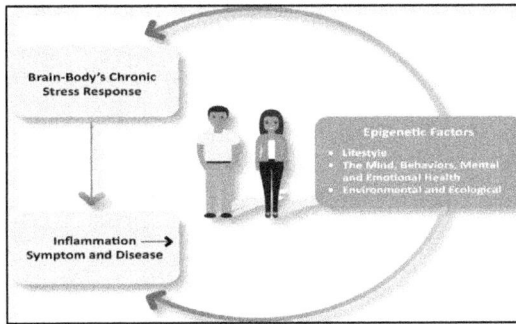

Figure 6. Other Influencing Factors of Stress of Inflammation

To change the way you feel, you have to make changes too, so start simply with day-to-day lifestyle like diet, movement, nature, and such (Chapter 7).

Then involve your mind.

Chronic illness = chronic stress to the body, it also = chronic stress to the mind too and vice versa.

> *Chronic illness = chronic body stress = chronic mind stress*
> *Chronic illness = chronic mind stress = chronic body stress*

So always make sure you include yourself and your behavior as part of any effective treatment plan (Chapter 8).

Just as your DNA is predetermined, your upbringing is too, and it has a tangible effect on behavior and how you form close relationships. This means that upbringing can impact health and serves as another factor you can decide to address within your treatment plan (Chapter 9).

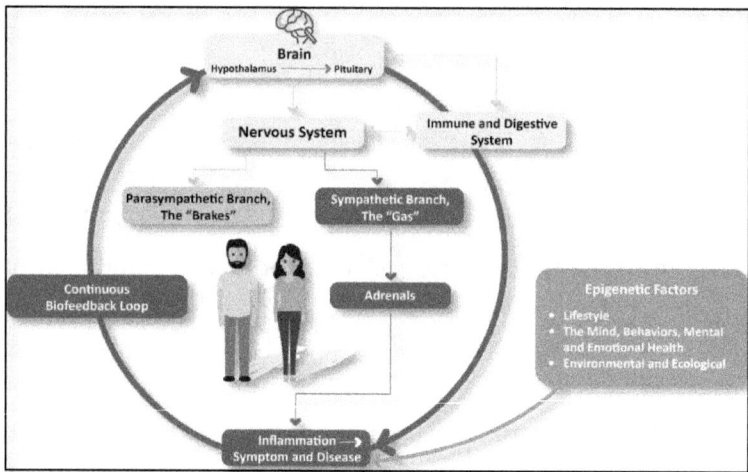

Figure 8. Putting it all Together

Chronic illness = chronic stress to the body and the mind too, which are all constantly interacting within your environment. Your mind-body associates traumas into your DNA, but it does the same with awesome, peak experiences too. Call upon those memories. Call upon all you have got, all you can control and put into your surroundings, into your own healing community, to create your own pharmhouse – your own community (Chapter 10).

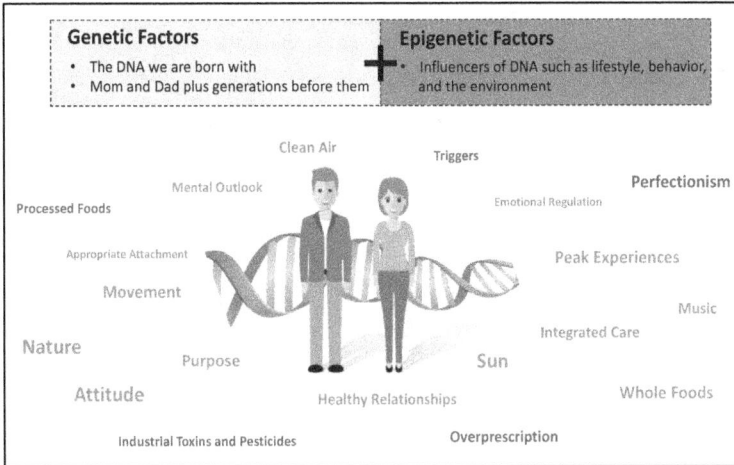

Figure 7. Creating your own Community

All of this has led us to a more simplified understanding of what an effective chronic illness treatment plan would look like – no matter what it is:

1) **Testing**
   - Assesses the body and mind with objective markers from the beginning and throughout

2) **Reset and Restore**
   - Two underlying factors for all chronic illnesses
   - *Reset* by less gas and less stress with more brakes, and more relaxing
   - *Restore* by reducing inflammation

3) **Lifestyle**
   - Incorporate epigenetic influencers of DNA

- Core needs like food, water, air, and movement are universal to every body

4) Involve Yourself

- Another epigenetic influencer of DNA
- From basic changes in habits and behaviors to upbringings and close relationships – make everything a part of the solution

5) Build a Community

- The last major epigenetic influencer on DNA
- Assemble a team and create your own pharmhouse, turning your environment into its own therapy

6) Press Play

- Adapt, readapt, and know you *will* get better

Quite simply, your treatment plan is effective if you get better. And you *can* get better. No matter the illness, the science continues to prove that we all have a genuine opportunity to be well.

Chapter 12: Press Play

As you put together and play out your treatment plan, your guide is how you feel. The factors of health – *your* factors of health – will either come together to help you feel better or they will cause you illness and struggle.

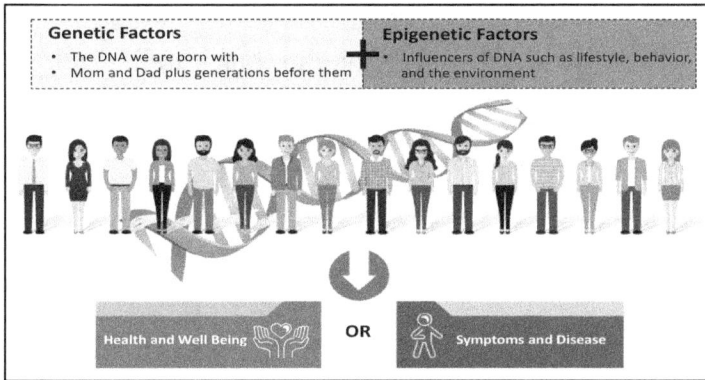

Figure 1. Factors of Health and Illness

The higher the body's score, the more this combination isn't working out for our health and well-being – the more we are struggling and swimming upstream against our DNA. Conversely, the lower the score, the better we feel, the higher our quality of life – and the more in alignment we are with our DNA, with who we are.

"When did this all start?" our intake nurse asked Jennifer.

"It began with sleep issues, but nothing crazy," the 28-year old teacher replied. The symptom would seemingly come out of nowhere and would last for a few days, but ultimately would resolve by week's end.

"It got a lot worse though after I changed grade levels." Then she got Covid and developed fatigue. She went to her primary doctor and they told her to take some time off from work to try and get some extra rest and recover. She did, but it didn't help. Her brain felt like it was constantly moving – going, going, going, yet her body was just exhausted.

This went on for two years. By the time she arrived at our center she had seen eight doctors, endured countless treatments and theories, and she was worse than ever.

"My primary thought was that it might be long Covid but he ended up referring me to an endocrinologist because of something in my hormones. Then after a while, they told me to see a psychologist – that it was in my head."

Step 1: Testing

Use testing to reveal the predictable biological patterns of chronic illness. Keep an especially keen eye on the body's impact from chronic stress and inflammation (Reset and Restore).

In addition to using labs to measure the impact on the body, you should also include additional standardized assessments and tests such as anxiety and depression screenings where anyone under 65 should be screened regularly.

Be sure to keep up with your standard physicals and exams alongside these mentioned lab values and psychological assessments.

Reset Pattern

We are looking for things here to gauge the impact that stress and the gas pedal have impacted the body. It will be there for every body and every illness. For Jennifer she had an elevated heart rate, elevated blood pressure, as well as a low ACTH, a brain hormone involved in the chronic stress pathway. An anxiety screening came back severe.

Restore Pattern

Here we are looking for things to gauge the impact that inflammation has had on the body. This includes overall inflammatory values as well as the impact the chronic stress response and inflammation have had on other aspects of the body such as the immune system, digestive, system, and adrenal glands. It's important to dampen the fight or flight response, but it's equally important to address the effect this response has had on the entirety of the brain-body.

Inflammation was widespread for Jennifer. She had impacts noted on her liver (hepatitis), her red blood cells (the cells that help carry oxygen and energy to cells), as well as inflammatory effects on the immune system. At 28, her sugar was now elevated to prediabetic levels – elevated liver enzymes, glucose, HbA1c, and CD8 T cells.

Step 2: Reset and Restore

"I don't feel like I ever really slept all that well," Jennifer said. "Then the fatigue and brain fog happened after that."

Her husband then glanced over to her, and she quickly looked back at me and said, "I also suffer from panic attacks."

Jennifer's body was clearly stressed and inflamed and her mind was too. The mind-body can't heal if it's stuck on the gas – much of its self-healing pathways can only be activated by its brake system. It also can't heal if half of its energy is already earmarked, putting out inflammatory fires throughout the brain-body.

Start by helping the body heal from these two underlying factors of all chronic illness. Start with the ingrained DNA that we all have in common. We need the body's help if we are going to have a shot at getting better. Every other therapy utilized will work better if this step is done first.

Reset Plan

By the time we saw Jennifer, I was able to patent our testing methods and the system used to formulate an IV and botanical regimen for our patients. We were able to customize formulations for how much brake chemistry and antioxidants were needed for the brain-body based on individual symptoms, labs, and vital signs.

I encourage you to find your way of getting things calmed down – your own brake therapies. Whether it be seeing other providers, taking a medication, and even ways of life – whatever helps you encourage your body to hit the brakes and lay off the gas. Without the brakes – without a calm nervous system – any treatment plan is literally fighting against a biological road block to get better.

Jennifer's labs necessitated lots of brake chemicals such as magnesium, taurine, and theanine. We also used a blend of botanicals that help with the same with herbs like passionflower, valerian, and lavender. After her third treatment, we layered in diaphragmatic breathing – another brake therapy – to help reinforce calming things down.

How do you know if you have Reset and gotten out of fight or flight?

You won't be as reactive – little stressors won't bother you as much, you won't be triggered as much – symptoms of anxiety, tension, pain, and sleep tend to improve, and you will be in more control.

How did we know Jennifer was beginning to calm things down?

She told us.

After 6 weeks, her elevated heart rate and blood pressure came down to healthy levels. Her chronic stress values improved, and her anxiety screening went from severe to low. She also hadn't had any panic attacks for the last four weeks and was sleeping an average of seven hours each night.

Restore Plan

As the body moves towards a Reset, it's equally as important to heal the downstream effects of the chronic stress response as well as any other inflammatory effects noted throughout the brain-body. You can't just address the nervous system and ignore that it's connected to our breathing, our heart rate, our immune and digestive systems, and so forth.

The inflammation noted in Jennifer's labs necessitated antioxidants that were incorporated simultaneously into her IV as well as into her botanical regimen with ingredients like glutathione, n-acetyl-cysteine, resveratrol, and quercetin, among others.

We also incorporated a group of botanicals, known as adaptogens – herbs that literally adapt to the environment they are in – to help Jennifer restore her adrenal health. Steroid medications or brain boosting supplements can support the adrenals too, but they also hit the gas pedal. Adaptogens can support the adrenals without hitting the gas. Additional adaptogens have also been shown to support the immune system while you can help to reduce inflammation in the digestive tract by incorporating healthy fibers, fermented foods, and botanicals like peppermint, licorice, and ginger.

As Jennifer worked her way through her treatment plan, nearly all of the noted inflammatory effects improved and she was no longer considered pre-diabetic. This coincided with vast improvements in her energy, anxiety, and sleep.

Step 3: Lifestyle

Parts III-VI of your Treatment Plan doesn't need to be done in any particular order. Once you have some baseline testing and you have begun to dampen the body's fight or flight response and reduce a little inflammation, you can move through these parts at your own pace and in no particular order. In other words, you don't have to wait to get the emotional therapy you need because you haven't finished addressing your diet yet. Work on whatever you can control. Epigenetic factors literally shape our DNA into helping us get better or keeping us sick. Lifestyle is the factor that has to meet the foundational needs of your body, of every body.

Diet, Exercise, and Breathing, Nature and Stress

In Jennifer's case, she was already eating pretty well. Her endocrinologist had recommended eating more whole foods and easing up on the caffeine which she had stuck with for the last two years. We just recommended more berries for the antioxidants and meal prepping to ease the day-to-day of cooking.

She had gotten away from exercise. She was just too tired to get to the gym, so we incorporated a light walk to get some movement going again. We also recommended a cheat meal, where Jennifer could eat her beloved pastries a couple times a week.

Alongside simple diet and exercise changes, our breathing serves as an everyday opportunity to improve oxygenation, bolster the brakes, and help us heal.

Stress causes breathing to predictably move away from the primary focuses of breathing like the diaphragm and nose and into compensatory aspects of the brain-body such as the mouth, ribcage, chest, and shoulders.

Diaphragmatic breathing hits the brakes while reinforcing healthy breathing to better maximize the 20,000 breaths we take per day. You can try this by simply laying down on your back with your knees bent, with one hand on your chest and one of your upper abdomen. In diaphragmatic breathing, only your hand on your abdomen should move as you slowly inhale and exhale through your nose. You can also try pursed lip breathing, where instead of slowly exhaling through your nose, you exhale through pursed lips – like blowing a kiss. Or box breathing, where you inhale for 4 seconds, hold for 4, exhale for 4, and pause for 4 seconds. Any of these breathing exercises can be done seated. You get the point – *Just Breathe* – [and buy Nestor's *Breath* if you don't believe me.]

Step 4: Involve your Mind

Without accepting any accountability and responsibility for your illness, you also handcuff your ability to help yourself. In part, it's like giving some of your power away – giving away the influence your mind and its behaviors can have on your illness.

While it can be hard to accept ownership over genetics you didn't choose and upbringings within environments that you had no say in – they are still your symptoms, your choices, your life.

Jennifer did her best to remain positive throughout the 4-year battle with her symptoms, but it had taken an emotional toll on her and her husband. They had been trying to get pregnant and remained unsuccessful for three years running.

> Chronic illness = chronic body stress = chronic mind stress
> Chronic illness = chronic mind stress = chronic body stress
> Feeling, sensations, thoughts → memories

Therapy allowed Jennifer to identify how she felt throughout her illness and see how this affected her relationship with her husband as well as shaped her thoughts and beliefs throughout the last four years. It gave her more of an understanding of how emotions and thoughts must be involved in her health and healing, a necessary skillset she can apply for the rest of her life.

Step 5: Build a Community

"I don't like meditation," Jennifer stated.

"Me neither," Tammy said back to Jennifer. Tammy had been practicing massage therapy and teaching meditation classes for close to 30 years. For Jennifer this was her first time with any sort of therapy like this and Tammy wanted to teach her in a small group outside at the pharmhouse.

"This isn't meditation," she continued, "You are just focusing your thoughts, your mind, on doing a conscious head-toe scan – almost like you're checking in on your body.

"I don't know, she said.

"Just try it, it'll help you get out of that head of yours for a bit."

Jennifer ended up really enjoying it and mindfulness as part of her nightly routine just before her bedtime prayers. She was starting to feel better *and* establish a healthy routine for herself to keep on that track.

Do all that you can to promote a positive influence on your DNA, a healthy environment around you. Create your own pharmhouse.

Step 6: Press Play

Jennifer made her way through six weeks of treatment, but not without setbacks – she had a panic attack at the end of her second week of treatment. In the fourth week, she didn't sleep for two days in a row, and she had struggles gauging her energy almost daily.

Sometimes your treatment plan will feel like two steps forward and one step back where the healing trajectory is rarely straightforward or linear. Despite how discouraging and frustrating pullback may feel, you will lose some battles. You don't need to win every battle to win the war.

Jennifer worked herself through the ups and downs of getting well. She began to gauge her improvement as week over week, month over month as opposed to day-to-day, moment to moment. Her labs improved right alongside her progress and as she stood there in the doorway on her last day of treatment, I knew she had turned the corner.

"I think I'm going to be okay," she said as I looked up from my desk, "No," she paused, "I know I am."

In the years since, Jennifer hasn't had a single panic attack, works full time and loves it – and she and her husband are enjoying every moment, passing this influence on to their now 3-year-old son.

Chapter 13: The Quest for a Cure versus Quality of Life

What is a cure?

Is it labs that improve, bacteria and viruses that get eradicated, diseases that can no longer be measured?

If a disease is cured, are the lasting effects of the disease cured, too?

The quest to cure chronic illness has led to the discovery of multiple different underlying causes. There are both predetermined genetic factors – that we are born with, as well as epigenetics factors – that we have more control over, influencers of genes like our lifestyle, our behaviors, and our environment.

Perception also plays an important role in health. The body is constantly perceiving itself on the inside and everything happening around it on the outside. And we can also have our own view of things, and sometimes that view is different from the body's. The choices we make throughout our life compound to either support our health or contribute to illness.

This relative nature of health and illness, means that sometimes the cure for your illness is different from the cure for your quality of life. It also means that there will be aspects of both that only you can cure. This was never more evident to me then when Tod walked into my office.

Adopted from ALS News Today[7], "A former soccer coach and military veteran, Tod had been working in accounting for several years when he began having trouble moving the fingers of his left hand. Originally thought to be a trigger finger that required surgery, Tod was stunned when he learned he had ALS. At the time, he was 59 years old.

When I first met Tod in the Spring of 2021, his symptoms had worsened and spread to his legs. He had pain and fatigue, trouble tying his shoes, and developed foot drop — difficulty lifting the front of his foot when walking.

After running extensive tests on Tod's body chemistry, we treated him with a six-week regimen of intravenous and contrast therapy — repeated exposure to cold and heat — and an oral botanical regimen. We also changed his diet and prescribed occupational therapy, acupuncture, and functional and neurological exercises.

After just a few short weeks, Tod slowed and even reversed some of the clinical findings as well as reporting a significant decrease in pain and an increase in his energy levels.

He displayed marked improvement in standardized occupational and functional testing in sensory awareness, body awareness, and weight shifting where obvious improvements in how he was walking were noted.

Tod agreed with that clinical evaluation.

"My mobility increased because of the occupational therapy. I got dexterity and mobility back in my hand. After working with my therapist, my stability and balance issues were better," Tod said, adding that he credited an "almost immediate" reduction in hand and joint pain to diet changes.

"My wife and I walked out of that [initial] meeting and we were both crying because there was a hope for a quality of life that we didn't have before, a better outlook, a better outcome."

He felt so much better that, on the day of his daughter's wedding, he was able to dress himself in his tuxedo, tie his shoes and necktie, walk his daughter down the aisle, and dance with her at the reception. He then was able to join his family on a post-wedding trip to Rome, Italy, where they went on an extensive walking tour.

"It was absolutely amazing," he said. "I felt pretty good for the most part, though the gluten-free diet went out the window. I did 25,000 to 30,000 steps a day. I was feeling good."

At his 12-month checkup, Tod's left hand had lost some function. Still, many improvements were retained, especially those pertaining to blood analyses, balance, breathing, and everyday function.

"I think it was the focus on repairing the body, based on the blood work pre-treatment and post-treatment, that caused the massive improvement in my body's function and also how physiologically I'm able to move," he said.

"I have to accept that I'm not going to referee a soccer match anytime soon, but my wife and I got out on the pickle court the other day and had a great time. These treatments allowed me to dance with my daughter at her wedding, which was probably the most special thing that I experienced in my life."" *~Adopted from ALS News Today*[7]

The large majority of chronic illnesses remain incurable which includes every neurodegenerative condition like Tod's. There's no single genetic anomaly that we have found thus far that is the underlying cause for Alzheimer's or Bipolar or Crohn's disease, like there is for that of Down's Syndrome or Cystic Fibrosis.

Chronic illness involves multiple brain-body systems, multiple contributory factors, involving multiple genes and interactions of those genes. And until all of these aspects are identified and cured – the focus needs to center around quality of life.

A model around quality of life allows for treating any contributory factor to the illness, even if it isn't the cure. The science shows there are therapies for your body and mind along with simple choices you can make that *will* improve your illness. Ultimately, the science shows that everyone can get better.

Even the simplest therapies and changes can help you improve. Posture, diet, and grounding have all been shown to decrease pain and reduce inflammation. Even things like happy thoughts and flossing your teeth have been shown to improve heart disease while exercising later in life reduces your risk of ever struggling with motor diseases like Parkinson's.

The National Institute of Health has shown that a healthier diet can improve your mental health. That eating more antioxidants or incorporating more healthy fatty acids like fish oils or avocados, can help improve symptoms for Parkinson's and ALS. It's even been shown that improving smell, hearing, or vision with therapies like hearing aids, glasses, and inhalation can improve cognition, memory, and reduce symptoms of dementia.

Maybe you can't cure your fatigue, your balance, your pain, your illness, but you can most certainly feel better. In fact, this type of model necessitates looking at each contributory factor, any possible aspect of the illness that could help us improve our condition, our quality of life.

Science and mainstream medicine have been slow to adopt a holistic model for healthcare as well as effective natural practices in part because of all its associated pseudoscience claims.

Yet, there are botanical formulations that are thousands of years old that continue to serve as standalone solutions in healthcare models around the world. In Japan, 148 botanical formulations are used for care while in China, traditional Chinese medicine goes right alongside conventional medicine as one solution.

It's similar in India where Ayurveda, yoga, and modern medicine are one healthcare system, and like that of Japanese and Chinese medicine, have well established botanical formulations, arts of movement, meditations, and entire medical philosophies and systematic methodologies. All of which view the body, its systems, and the mind as one cohesive unit. They have all employed these truths as medicine for at least thousands of years.

In America we are slowly adopting that the mind-body are inseparable, that a holistic integrated model is in fact the most effective treatment model for chronic illness because, as physicist Fritjof Capra concludes in his New York Times Best Selling Book, *The Tao of Physics,* – we essentially have to prove today's science around science that has already existed for thousands of years[8].

For modern medicine, these scientific truths are still recent. It took until 1991 to determine the nervous system was connected to the immune system and vice versa. It took until 2015, to really consider the "gut-brain" connection. We now know that neurons are spread everywhere throughout the brain-body, that we have trillions of cells and even more connections between those cells. We now know that behaviors do matter, lifestyle choices add up, and the mind and body act unequivocally as one unit.

It wasn't until even more recently, that science has been able to track DNA changes over time, over generations of people. It revealed that any one of us can be working with not just years of habits and influencers, but decades and in some cases centuries of erosive choices and traumatic influences to our DNA. The research showed that ultimately the culmination of your choices or the traumatic events in your life will leave lasting impressions on your DNA and your kids' DNA and their kids' too. Heck, the body still holds onto the memory of the bubonic plague all these centuries later, let alone the dangers of war or a genocide of human betrayal.

The DNA we are born with is from our ancestors. This includes any chronic illness they experienced and the circumstances surrounding them. It includes any traumatic experiences as well as the culmination of their behaviors and day-to-day lifestyle choices. The health of the body and mind of everyone before you, will directly impact the foundation you have, the DNA you are born with.

It can't, however, predetermine your path. Our DNA is a culmination of both what we are born with and how we decide to influence it. We do the best with what we have, striving to make a better life for our kids, for the next generation. As the generations go by, the science continues to help us become more aware of the information surrounding health and illness – granting us the opportunity to change it.

Providing a better life for our kids comes through providing them a better opportunity for health than we had. To provide them less struggle in their mind and less disease in their body. As a parent, you are solely responsible for the epigenetic influence on your kids' DNA – for their lifestyle, their behavior, and their environment.

If you knew finding the cure for your quality of life would make your kids healthier, would you look for it?

What if you knew not changing your lifestyle or addressing your inflammation would not only make you sicker, but that it would cause your kid's DNA to be sicker too? Would you then make the change?

No one would ever want to experience some of the diseases and sufferings that are ever present in our world. Nor would we ever wish it or think that we are passing these burdens to our own kids.

No kid, no parent, no person should have that type of burden, the burden of disease that people like Tod are expected to carry, and the countless more like him. A single 30-minute doctor's visit to learn of his rapidly progressing, incurable condition, where 80% of individuals are gone within two to four years. A single doctor's visit that turned his entire world upside down.

Tod works so hard and knows despite any effort, he will continue to worsen. He knows that despite any effort, influences, changes, and more – the effect of his treatment plan will always trend downwards. It is unfair.

He didn't eat well all the time, he has trauma, he worked too much, but is that any different from you or me? All of our bodies age, none of us are perfect, all of us have thoughts as voices in our head, and we all get sick.

How is it that some are predisposed to autoimmunity, cancer, and neurodegeneration while others have heart disease or diabetes, and some seemed spared altogether?

There are, in fact, positive genetic predispositions too – the exact opposite of generational trauma. That instead of trauma of stress, abuse, war, and genocide – an environment and its people help foster health and well-being, passing *that influence* down. We call them blue zones, and they are communities around the world that people consistently live healthier and longer. Where generational wealth is generational health.

They aren't doing anything overly special – people in blue zones make healthy day-to-day lifestyle choices, keep themselves moving, have stable environments, and surround themselves with healthy relationships – all the while living in the same world as you and me.

This is what they pass down – healthy choices, healthy behaviors – healthy influences on DNA. They've just been doing it day in and day out for generations and generations.

Instead of passing down a lifetime of unhealthy choices or insufferable traumas, they pass down an opportunity of health that comes built in with positive influences and peak life experiences – to make the health and wellbeing of the next generation a little easier.

How different the opportunity of health is for all of us. Some of us have had relatives that were literally wiped out through genocide and war. Some have had their ancestors enslaved in the ultimate act of human betrayal. Some are still dealing with this today, watching missiles fly and their homes reduced to rubble, wondering what will become of them, of their kids.

Is it the luck of the birthright? To be born into a stable government and out of poverty? To be born with healthy and loving parents? A trauma free family tree?

In the end, to have a genetic predisposition for conditions like Alzheimer's or ALS means that your family before you has endured a lot of pain, suffering, and illness. It means that for whatever reasons, the epigenetic influencers have compounded into enough generational trauma to predispose your DNA to some of the worst conditions that exist. That even if your own choices are perfect in your own life, your ancestry predisposes you to great pain and suffering regardless.

Should you just give up? Should Tod give up? What is health and happiness at this point? When you know you can't get escape the fate of your body. What is quality of life then, when you know can't cure the body, the illness?

The largest study ever completed on happiness came out with only one conclusion. Beginning in 1938 and lasting over multiple generations, the 85-year Harvard study found that have strong relationships are the most significant source of happiness. That despite the peaks and valleys of successes and failures, of good health or serious illness – "positive relationships allow us to be happier, healthier, and help us live longer."[9]

That, although we may never cure our body of the illness, we can be still be happy – *that we are still in control of our quality of life.*

As hundreds of millions of Americans and billions of others worldwide continue to suffer from chronic illnesses, we can all do more to ease that burden on ourselves, our kids, and our fellow humans – to make a path towards quality of life easier and more realistic for one lifetime.

Work to nurture your nature, not fight against it. It starts with being a better teammate to your body and by recognizing we should relax a bit and lay off the gas. That pleading ignorance around core needs like food and movement is no longer an excuse.

We also need to acknowledge ourselves as part of the problem so we can become part of the solution. There is no fault by accepting ownership, or by accepting help.

It is true that the help needs more help too. There is such a significant shortage of healthcare workers, with an average of 10-20 minutes spent per visit on illnesses that often involve years, if not decades of one's life. On top of that, access to any form of integrative holistic care exists primarily in emergency medicine, at universities, or inpatient treatment programs where it needs to trickle down and replace the primary care level if we are ever going to make any real change.

While guidelines exist regarding illness, mental health, and lifestyle, family and primary care can do more by establishing standardized assessments of these guidelines as well as establishing more expansive and consistent baseline testing to gauge people year over year.

The testing needs improvement too, especially with early testing and prevention. These conditions are forming well before we feel them and even longer before we get diagnosed.

By the time we do get a diagnosis, it often quickly leads to drugs. So often, in fact, that an estimated 60 million Americans are overprescribed their medications. While drugs can be an instrumental tool in an effective treatment plan, they can't shoulder the entire load of chronic illness, nor do they represent all the senses and stimuli the body can use as medicine.

And while the science, doctors, and patients continue to inevitably move in that direction, insurance continues to do its own thing. Have you been to a restaurant and gotten the bill for $20 and then only paid $10 and left? Or only pay $50 for your $100 grocery bill? No one in their right mind would do so. Yet, that's insurance, they get charged 4x what is appropriate for the services and pay what they want, as if the entire system is negotiating our healthcare, like bartering for a t-shirt on vacation.

Instead of battling to reduce costs or improve access, or fighting on different sides of germ versus terrain, alternative versus conventional, eastern versus western – aren't we all on the same team? Aren't we all just trying to feel better?

It shouldn't be good enough to any of us for these constraints to continue to negatively impact our health. It shouldn't be good enough for billions of people to be sick each and every day, for that influence to be passed down and inevitably be the fate of the next generation. We all deserve the opportunity of a blue zone, a genuine opportunity of health.

You have to look at the health of your parents and want to do better for the sake of yourself. You have to look at your kids and know that giving them a healthy lifestyle, secure behavior, and a stable environment will make them healthier and more resilient to disease. And that in doing so you are literally getting better and leaving the next generation healthier than when you left it. That's what we all strive for isn't it? A life where our kids have every opportunity to be healthy and happy.

It's now been nearly four and a half years since Tod's diagnosis and over four years since we treated him. While he had some remarkable progress in the first eighteen months following treatment, the disease has continued to progress over the last few years. Tod is largely wheelchair bound now. He struggles a lot, but he still is able to enjoy his friends and family. Tod is also a grandfather now when 80% of people with his disease are no longer with us.

So, I'll ask again – what is a cure? What is your cure?

Is it labs improving, diseases that can no longer be measured? Is it freedom, happiness? Is a cure the only thing that can help you feel better?

Only you can answer that.

Chapter 14: The DNA of Health

Regardless of your circumstances, at some point your health will be up to you. Which treatments are most appropriate for you? What does calm even mean? What should I do first with my diet? How do I even go about changing certain behaviors? Do I do all these things at once?

The understanding of all that goes into chronic illness can only take you so far without having to actually integrate this understanding into our life. Without eventually having to press play.

So, what can you do to get better *right now*?

Whatever is in your control.

You'll need to start with some changes if you are going to change the way you feel. Begin with any of the three major epigenetic factors of DNA, something you do each and every day. Start with small adjustments and make them consistent. The changes you are making today won't be felt tomorrow.

> ### Simplified Diet and Movement Recommendations:
>
> - Eat more whole foods, less processed ones, and drink filtered water
> - Incorporate easy means of veggies, fruits, fibers, and antioxidants into smoothies, overnight oats, or chia pudding for a simple snack or meal
> - Incorporate healthy fats, slower digesting carbs, and adequate protein
> - Maximize high fiber foods, minimize sugar, and diversify foods
> - Severe illnesses should avoid allergen prone food like gluten, dairy and eat smaller, simple, and more frequent meals throughout the day
> - Try and get some form of movement in every day
> - Start with light movement like a short walk
> - Over time, work to sweat and challenge your body and mind
> - Try elevating movement's healing potential with targeted rehab or exercises or arts of movement like yoga, tai chi, or qi gong

Lifestyle can be broken down into a few fundamental aspects.

- The food we eat
- The water we drink
- The air we breathe, and
- How much we move, or exercise.

By no means do you need to be perfect, nor incorporate each and every step. Just do what you can to move in the right direction, day in and day out.

At a minimum,

- Drink Filtered Water
  - o Whole house filter, drinking water filter, bottled
- Eat More Whole Foods and Less Processed Ones
  - o More out of your fridge and less out of a wrapper
- Exercise
  - o A walk will do, any movement will do
- Get Outside More
  - o Make the environment part of your lifestyle
- Breathe
  - o Filters and Purifiers, Diaphragmatic Breathing

You can install a whole house water filter, buy a Berkey, or grab a water filter at the grocery store, but you need to drink filtered or purified water. The same goes for the air inside your house. Pollution accounts for millions of deaths each year, and simply keeping your home's air quality clean can go a long way to keeping you healthy. You can filter it with your HVAC, or simply get a few HEPA filters on Amazon for the primary rooms of your home. Use less plastic and avoid unnecessary chemicals where you can.

Make sure you combine healthy air with healthy breathing.

> ### Diaphragmatic Breathing
>
> - Lay down on your back on a flat surface with your knees bent. You can use a pillow(s) under your head or your knees if needed.
> - Place one hand on your upper chest and one hand on your upper belly (just below your ribcage)
> - As you slowly inhale through your nose, only the hand on your belly should move, while the hand on your chest should remain still
> - Exhale through your nose and let your belly relax and fall inward
> - Repeat this process for about 15 min, several times per day if possible

You can use your routine for breathing as an opportunity to start creating your own pharmhouse, your own healthy healing environment. From smells, sights, sounds, and people, make sure your home is a place you want to be.

And do what you can to bring the outdoors, in. Nature itself is healing, where people who are raised with more trees and more greenspace experience less disease and less mental health issues. A room could be your pharmhouse, your backyard could be too.

You can be too.

Acknowledge yourself as part of this. You aren't to blame or at fault, but it is your life and you are absolutely responsible and accountable for your health. You *will* have setbacks, but you *will* get better too. Make sure your behavior is part of the solution.

These same very changes also ensure you are doing your part too. Restore your body and not add to the inflammation you are already experiencing. For example, eating more whole foods, reducing processed ones, and eating more antioxidants, all serve as ways to reduce inflammation and improve lifestyle's impact on your DNA.

In order to ensure these efforts aren't wasted, the body's roadblock to healing must be removed. You have to get your body calm and Reset. This can come by way of any therapy or activity that reduces stress and promotes the body's brake system, such as meditation, sleep, yoga, breathing and more.

There are so many factors that went into your illness and your treatment plan needs to address all of them. As you begin to incorporate these changes, chances are you'll need some help to adequately address these factors as well as deeper routed aspects of your lifestyle, behavior, and environment.

So, what can you do with your Doctor, *right now?*

You can start by getting on an optimal medication and/or supplement regimen. We all want to be medication and pill free but chances are if you have chronic illness you just can't avoid doing something here.

You need therapies that are short term solutions – ones that work now – while filling in long term solutions right alongside. This is where medications are best served in an effective treatment plan. It's okay to treat symptoms if you're also addressing the causes too.

While MDs and DOs can help us with these regimens and various other factors of chronic illness, so can countless other healthcare practitioners.

Psychologists have been well documented to significantly impact behavior and relationships while acupuncture has been shown to positively affect many chronic symptoms including fatigue, anxiety, insomnia, pain, and hormonal disorders, among others.

In additional to helping from a chemical perspective, sometimes employing chiropractors can help with the structural and mechanical factors of the illness. As can massages, myofascial, lymphatic drainage, and cranial-sacral therapy too.

Physical and occupational therapists can improve strength, flexibility, and mobility while arts of meditation and movement like yoga, Pilates, and qi gong have been documented to consistently reduce stress, improve energy and improve overall well-being.

Naturopathic doctors spend their whole careers studying and implementing natural healthcare solutions and even within conventional medicine, we can employ multiple MD specialties ranging from neurology, endocrinology, and immunology and more.

At a minimum,

- Gather testing
    - Baseline starting point and checkpoint follow ups
- Get some help
    - Assemble your team, you don't need to fight alone
- Get the *appropriate help*
    - Match your symptoms with the right professionals

You aren't a bad person because you need help. You aren't a bad person in admitting you need help. We all need help.

Even if it seems unobtainable, start working towards,

- A Stable Environment
    - Healing only occurs on a stable foundation

- Work-Life Balance
  - Health>Relationships>Money
- Building your own Pharmhouse
  - Immerse yourself in getting better
- Healthier Relationships
  - Arguably the most important factor for happiness

It's okay to be sick. Yes, our healthcare system struggles with chronic illness. Yes, it should be more holistic, more accessible, far less expensive and frankly – more effective. But you can't stay sick. At least not anymore, the science shows that we can and will get better.

Simply said…

Chronic Illness Treatment Plan

1) Testing
   - Assesses the body and mind with objective markers from the beginning and throughout
2) Reset and Restore
   - Two underlying factors for all chronic illnesses
   - *Reset* by less gas and less stress with more brakes, and more relaxing
   - *Restore* by reducing inflammation
3) Lifestyle

- Incorporate epigenetic influencers of DNA
- Core needs like food, water, air, movement, and relaxing are universal to every body

4) Involve Yourself

- Another epigenetic influencer of DNA
- From basic changes in habits and behaviors to upbringings and close relationships – make everything a part of the solution

5) Build a Community

- The last major epigenetic influencer on DNA
- Assemble a team and create your own pharmhouse, turning your environment into its own therapy

6) Press Play

- Adapt, readapt, and know you *will* get better

Nobody sets out for a life with chronic illness, or worse yet, to pass that burden on to your kids. It's not that your ancestors chose this either. Generational trauma among ancestral trees act like ticking time bombs for anyone that is born. But nonetheless, it was their DNA, their life, their responsibility too. And those changes to their DNA are taken in, copied and passed on – to you.

Ultimately, the freedom of health is a privilege that is dictated by your body and given to you by your parents and their parents before them. We all deserve to be born into generational health instead of generational trauma. We all deserve to have our kids live in ancestral blue zones instead of geographical ones. Ultimately, we all deserve a genuine opportunity to be healthy.

It's up to you to seize that opportunity. Getting better is as much scientific as it is, you. Do your best. Take that extra walk. Eat the healthier lunch. Listen to your body a little bit more. Stress less where you can. Move towards people that love and support you and move away from those who don't. Just breathe. In the end, getting better is a lifestyle.

In the end, you *can* get better. No matter what, *Health is for Everybody.*

Appendix A: Chronic Illness Lab Panel

This is the panel needed for any chronic illness. If you have heart disease, chronic pain, Crohn's disease, arthritis, anxiety, fibromyalgia, depression, and so forth – this is the panel you need to start with.

Table 3: Chronic Illness Lab Panel

Lab Test	Ideal	High	Low	Notes
ACTH, pg/mL Adrenocorticotropin Hormone	20-30	>45	<13	High short-term stress Low with chronic stress
TSH, uIU/mL Thyroid Stimulating Hormone	<2.0	>4.0		High, the body needs more thyroid Low, thyroid is often ok
Prolactin, ng/dL	Varies, 5-20	>25	<4	Largely used as context for pituitary health
DHEA, ug/dL Dehydroepiandroster one	125-300M 100-175F	>375 >275	<100 <75	Indicator of Adrenals/Hormones Converts to testosterone
CBC w/ Differential* Complete Blood Cell Count White Blood Cells (WBCs)	5.5-7.5	>9.5	<4	Many important values, see notes WBCs along with T cells are good overall immune indicators
CD4/CD8 Ratio	1.8-2.2	>3.7	<1.5	T cell health Immune and Autoimmune Indicator
Ferritin, ng/mL	150-250M 50-100F	>350 M >150 F	<35 M/F	Essentially Iron Storage High = Inflammation

				Low = Malabsorption/Nutrient Deficiency
Free T3, pg/mL Free Active Thyroid	3-4.2	>4.5	<2.8	Pair with TSH and other hormones
Testosterone, ng/dL			<300M <15F	Use in context with other hormones. Females should test day 20-22 of cycle
Estradiol, pg/mL			<50M <80F	Use in context with other hormones. Females should test day 20-22 of cycle Estrone is another type of estrogen found elevated in males with hormone inflammation
Progesterone, ng/mL			<2F	Not necessary for Male. Females should test day 20-22 of cycle
CRP, mg/L C Reactive Protein	<2	>3	N/A	Inflammatory Risk, Cardiovascular
Homocysteine, umol/L	<10	>12		High = High Oxidative Stress, Low Glutathione
HbA1c, % Hemoglobin A1c		>5.5		Inflammatory Risk, Sugar, Cellular
CMP**, Complete Metabolic Panel Glucose, mg/dL AST, IU/L ALT, IU/L	75-90 15-28 15-30	>95 >35 >40	<2.8 <12 <12	Many important values, Glucose is your sugar AST and ALT are liver enzymes, measuring liver inflammation

*There are many other values that are important in a CBC including, red blood cells, MCHC, MCV the breakdown of white blood cells, and more

** There are many other values that are important in a CMP including kidney and bile values, other liver values, among others

Appendix B: Meds, Actions, and Equivalents

As with the rest of the book, this isn't medical advice. Meds are serious, so any changes need to be done with your doctor. This is just meant to show there are additional therapies and natural chemicals that may work in place or in complement.

Table 4: Meds, Actions, and Equivalents

Drug Type	Common Drugs	Action	Alternatives
Benzodiazepines	Xanax, Ativan, Clonazepam, Lorazepam, Temazepam	↓□	GABA, Theanine
Alcohol	All Types	↓□	GABA, Theanine, Adaptogens
Opiates and Opioids	Oxycontin, Oxycodone, Percocet, Vicodin, Heroin, etc	↓□	PT/OT, Injections, Grounding, CBT
Sleep Aids	Trazadone, Ambien, Lunesta	↓□	Magnesium, Taurine, 5-HTP, Valerian, Lavender, Chamomile, Theanine
Stimulants	Adderall, Vyvanse, Ritalin	↑□	Adaptogens like Maca, Rhodiola, Ginseng, Ashwagandha, Triphala, Astragalus
Steroids	Hydrocortisone, prednisolone	↑□	Adaptogens like Tulsi, Triphala, Ashwagandha, Astragalus
Anti-inflammatories	NSAIDS, non NSAIDS	↑□	Curcumin, Resveratrol, Quercetin, NAC, Glutathione

Works Cited

1) Van der Kolk, B. The Body Keeps the Score. Brain, Mind and Body in the Healing of Trauma. Penguin, 2014.

2) Garber, J., and Brownlee, S. Medication Overload: America's Other Drug Problem. Brookline, MA: The Lown Institute, 2019. DOI: https://doi.org/10.46241/LI.WOUK3548

3) Gupta, S. One Nation Under Stress. Documentary. HBO, 2019.

4) Nestor, J. Breath. Penguin Life, 2020.

5) Patrick, R. Senate Aging Commission. 14 February 2025.

6) Shirai T, Tsushita K. Lifestyle Medicine and Japan's Longevity Miracle. Am J Lifestyle Med. 2024 Mar 19;18(4):598-607. doi: 10.1177/15598276241234012. PMID: 39262888; PMCID: PMC11384843.

7) Chapman, M. *ALS Success Story Delivers Man's "Most Special Day."* ALS News Today, 2022, November 14. https://alsnewstoday.com/news/als-success-story-delivers-mans-most-special-day/

8) Capra, Fritjof. The Tao of Physics: An Exploration of the Parallels between Modern Physics and Eastern Mysticism. Shambhala, 1975.

9) Schultz, M., Waldinger, R. The Good Life: Lessons from the World's Longest Scientific Study of Happiness. Simon and Schuster, 2023.

www.ingramcontent.com/pod-product-compliance
Lightning Source LLC
LaVergne TN
LVHW051600080426
835510LV00020B/3069